REIKI HEALING: A MASTERCLASS

THE STEP-BY-STEP, COMPREHENSIVE GUIDE TO MASTER REIKI & HEALING MEDITATION FOR BEGINNERS

SIYA ISHANI

© **Copyright 2019 - All rights reserved.**

The content contained within this book may not be reproduced, duplicated or transmitted without direct written permission from the author or the publisher.

Under no circumstances will any blame or legal responsibility be held against the publisher, or author, for any damages, reparation, or monetary loss due to the information contained within this book. Either directly or indirectly.

Legal Notice:

This book is copyright protected. This book is only for personal use. You can't amend, distribute, sell, use, quote or paraphrase any part, or the content within this book, without the consent of the author or publisher.

Disclaimer Notice:

Please note the information contained within this document is for educational and entertainment purposes only. All effort has been executed to present accurate, up to date, and reliable, complete information. No warranties of any kind are declared or implied. Readers acknowledge that the author isn't engaging in the rendering of legal, financial, medical or professional advice. The content within this book has been derived from various sources. Please consult a licensed professional before attempting any techniques outlined in this book.

By reading this document, the reader agrees that under no circumstances is the author responsible for any losses, direct or indirect, which are incurred as a result of the use of information contained within this document, including, but not limited to, — errors, omissions, or inaccuracies.

INTRODUCTION

"Every house is built on a foundation, and the foundation of your body is your life force. If the Chi is unhealthy it will affect the physical aspects of your life and thus our Reiki system is the key to unlock this impediment to your progress."

Are you suffering? Have your Doctors, Psychologists, and Psychiatrists tried to talk or medicate you to "health". Have you seen little or no results? Well, that's not surprising…

In today's hectic world, more and more people are suffering with seemingly ever-increasing health issues. Issues with weight loss, or weight gain are great examples of our problem with modern medicine.

We meticulously plan out our diets and follow through with our exercise and see poor results. The math says that we've eaten this many calories, and burned that many calories, so we should be loosing weight, and yet we don't achieve our goals.

You might also have a significant other that you're having problems with, or that you'd just like to be closer to. Perhaps you've tried picnics in the park, dance lessons, and more, but yet you still both find yourself arguing at the over little things that shouldn't really matter.

An unhealthy Chi can lead to an unhealthy relationship. Reiki, especially when done by both members of a couple, can provide a tranquility of spirit that allows both members to relax and grow together in harmony, instead of growing slowly apart in discord.

Ailments such as arthritis, migraines, carpal tunnel and others can be alleviated with the proper allocation of Reiki healing in conjunction with your current medical regimen. Often pain is simply a symptom of an energy imbalance in the body, and Reiki is designed to address this very situation specifically.

Reiki Healing can also help with chronic fatigue or insomnia by addressing the inconsistencies in your energies that you might not even be consciously aware of. Do you notice periods where your physical energy waxes or wanes for no reason that you can attribute to diet or environment? Then the Reiki system laid out here could be the answer.

If you've been suffering from panic attacks or other forms of anxiety, and nothing the doctors have prescribed or the psychologists have had you 'talk out' seem to help, then consider adding Reiki to your medical regimen. Doctors don't generally subscribe to the fact that a disharmony of the life force can be just as important as medications or psychobabble. This leads to a treatment of *symptoms* while ignoring the *source*. Reiki can bring a balance to your treatment and may be the only thing that you need, but you won't know until you try it for yourself.

As we progress through this book, we'll discuss how and why this system WORKS, as well as giving you the tools, so that you learn and practice Reiki healing from the comfort of your own home. As you learn to manipulate your life-energies you'll soon find that you can have the results that medical science has failed to provide time and time again.

It's all about what you know.

There are a number of reasons that you've come to Reiki and we hope not to disappoint. Simply pursue this knowledge with patience, learn what you read, practice what you learn, and soon let what you've learned become what you truly know. The results that arise will make it worth your while.

Let's continue to Chapter 1 and begin preparing you for the bright future ahead!

1

WHY TRY OUR APPROACH TO REIKI HEALING?

You probably know that Reiki is an energy-healing system but do you know how it works?

The Chinese have a word called 'Chi', very similar to 'Prana' or 'life force' to the Hindus, and it's fundamental to the way that Reiki healing works. Chi is present in everything and pervades the universe. Think of it as personal energy resonating with the energy of the Universe.

Literally translating as 'air', like the air that you breathe in every day in order to sustain yourself. Believers in Chi, Prana, Auras and other concepts of life energy abound across the world and use this energy to their benefit. Not just practitioners looking for healing - many martial artists subscribe to the belief as well, using the energies to protect themselves or to improve the veracity of their attacks.

With Reiki, our concern is going to be utilizing the Chi for healing and harmony. As it travels through our body it employs body-highways known as meridians and knowing the location of these Meridians can empower you to heal many ailments quite quickly and quite successfully. We'll go into more about the Meridians and Reiki applications through them later.

In the Introduction we advised you of some issues that Reiki can assist you with. Here are a few more issues that Reiki can address *(Keep in mind, this is still just a taste of what you can learn to heal. Reiki can do all of these things, and more)*:

Reduction of stress levels in your life

Reiki healing creates not only harmony but a state of deep relaxation that can decrease stress factors in your life. Think about it in practical terms. Have you ever had to make a decision in an emergency? When you're relaxed then you're much more likely to make a sound, reasonable judgment call then when you're panicked or over-stimulated due to stress.

Increase the body's ability to heal itself from harm

Reiki works with your Chi energy, which when balanced, is said to improve your self-healing factor. When the body's life force is healthy this effect is only natural. Add is a little exercise and you'll find your body performing at peak capacity.

Help in cleansing the body of the toxins that we ingest each and every day

We ingest a surprising amount of toxins from day to day, often in the form of chemical additives or preservatives in products that might not be as '100% natural' as advertised. Reiki improves circulation and the body's ability to shed toxins, thus improving your overall health.

Stimulating creativity for those who wish to express themselves artistically or otherwise

When your energies are balanced through Reiki, you'll find yourself more receptive to the inspirations of your surroundings. A healthy Chi leads to less distractions and in such a state of harmonic bliss you'll find yourself better able to create.

Bolstering the immune system to fend off or fight sickness

As the body's energy is balanced with Reiki healing, the immune system steadily grows more efficient. This can lead to your body producing more white blood cells and giving your immune system a much-needed boost for a healthier life.

Intrigued? You're in good company. A 2007 study indicates that 1.2 million people in the United States alone have taken the time to explore the benefits that Reiki can provide them. This demonstrates a general unhappiness that the medical community alone has been insufficient to address. Thus, other measures are quite obviously required.

You're in the right place!

Our approach can help you to address these issues and many, many more.

So, are you ready to get started?

Great!

First we are going to discuss a little of the history of Reiki and then we'll get you started on some healing basics. You'll then start building your Reiki-toolbox with some new and powerful techniques as we go.

2

REIKI HISTORY PRIMER

What's the history behind Reiki? Well, Reiki originally hails from Japan, the brainchild of a man named Mikao Usui.*

Mr. Usui, a lay Monk (a non-clerical monk, who takes local vows but wasn't ordained), Mikao was living in a time in Japan's history when a wide variety of spiritual practices were commonplace, with Buddhism, Shinto, and Taoist beliefs being the primary modes of spirituality.

In the early 1920's (reportedly 1922) Mikao would have a profound spiritual revelation that he'd spend the last 4 years of his life sharing with the world.

Usui Reiki was born.

While containing Reiki healing techniques, the mass of Mikao's teachings amounted to quite a bit more, with philosophies and insights not only from Japanese traditions but from ancient Chinese medicine as well. Excited about his spiritual discovery, Mikao Usui travelled the length and breadth of Japan to spread his revelations, bringing students into the fold who shared his enthusiasm for this new system of ancient wisdoms.

While he taught more than 2000 students before he died, he had appointed only 16 of these to be Reiki Masters. One of the Masters, a retired Naval officer by the name of Chujiro Hayashi, received Mikao's blessing to open a clinic in Tokyo. Having worked extensively with Usui, Chijuro desired to take the healing aspects from the main body of Usui's teachings and make them more accessible to the general public.

From this, he developed his own style of Reiki, keeping meticulous notes as the 16 Masters at his clinic worked, leading to data in regards to which hand positions were most favorable for treatment. He also began imparting healing elements of Chinese medicine, such as Meridians, and Hindu elements such as Chakra points into his practice.

Chijuro, like his mentor, began training masters as well, and one of them would be a Japanese-American by the name of Hawayo Takata.

Hawayo had herself been healed from a number of ailments through Reiki treatment and, as such, became a devoted student of Sensei Hayashi.

Eventually she'd bring Reiki to Hawaii in 1937.

Eventually, she'd bring Reiki to the mainland United States.

During her life, she taught for 40 years before beginning the training of her own Reiki Masters, of which there were 22 at her time of death in 1980.

Modern Reiki has evolved but as it employs ancient wisdom at the core, much has stayed the same. While Takata's 22 Reiki Masters have spread her teachings and style, in this day and age a number of styles and combinations are practiced worldwide.

It just goes to show that Sensei Usui was on to something…

REIKI BASICS - THE PRINCIPLES, HOW IT WORKS, AND MERIDIANS

The 5 Principles of Reiki

1. *Just for today, do not be angry*
2. *Just for today, do not worry*
3. *Just for today, be grateful*
4. *Just for today, work hard*
5. *Just for today, be kind to others.*

While much of Mikao Usui's teachings were excised by Chijuro in favor of promoting strictly the healing precepts of Reiki, much of Miikao's teachings still remain. The 5 precepts of Reiki are one of these principles. These are words to live by, elegant in their simplicity, let's take a moment to contemplate this wisdom.

1. *Just for today, do not be angry.*

We get angry over the slightest things. Things that sometimes don't even matter in an hour or two, except as 'water cooler' talk (and what a state of things, when we tell stories of someone cutting us off in traffic and how angry we got, as if two ugly things suddenly have more merit then the beauty in life.)

Take a day off from your anger.

Take today off from your anger. When you feel it coming up, contemplate something that made you laugh, or something profound like the birth of your child, or even just distract yourself by trying to describe the smells around you in a mental dialogue. Try this little experiment and at the end of the day ask yourself, 'Was my day better or worse without the anger?'. Just something to contemplate.

2. Just for today, do not worry.

Worry does very little for us and quite a lot of things against us. Increased stress levels raise our blood pressure. Too much worry can promote anxiety or rash decisions. Try to turn that energy, if only for today, into either preparation or fuel for a more productive day. Another good alternative is rest, as the Vikings used to say, 'If you spend all night worrying about the battle, then you'll be tired in the morning when you must fight it.'

3. Just for today, be grateful.

It's amazing how often we can forget the things that we've in lieu of complaining about the things that we want. A roof, enough food, employment - these are things that people across the world and even close to your home simply don't have. Is it really worth your sense of peace to create a bad day for yourself and others just because they left the onions off your sandwich at a restaurant or your friend gave you a Pepsi instead of a Coke?

You have your health and a full belly, you're already ahead of the game and from a practical standpoint, time spent feeling ungrateful is time you could be spending writing that best-selling novel, painting that new work everyone will marvel at, prototyping your genius invention, or planning that amazing small business. When you catch yourself (and sometimes it's easy to forget), stop yourself from being ungrateful. Try it, just for today.

4. Just for today, work hard.

One of life's little-known and oft forgotten pleasures and treasures is the feeling that you get from a job well-done. We get lost in our daily routine and after awhile it seems like we are running on autopilot. While you might feel tempted to just fly through the day like a robot, why not take the time, assert your will and your power of self, and show them just what you've got? Oddly enough, this simple precept gives you a way to break out of your routine while you're in the middle of experiencing it. Just for today, let it be your first day at work, give it your all and see how you feel when it's behind you. You may be pleasantly surprised.

5. Just for today, be kind to others.

Sometimes the world seems to move at the speed of light. We

feel like we need to push ahead, streak past whatever is in our path, and get it all behind us. The problem with this is that it's an attitude towards time, rather than an attitude towards the world. When we push and rush we tend to find ourselves being rude to others. When we assume that every homeless person is simply out for a drink, then we sometimes consign good people to hunger while we starve our own souls in the process.

Slow down.

Today, be kind. Feed the birds. Give the dog an extra treat. Give the homeless guy some change. Offer your sibling the last pancake. There is an endless list of little things that you can do to be kinder and every little bit makes the universe that much better. Just for today, don't take, but give.

HOW IT WORKS

Now that you've had a taste of the philosophy, let's get to the reason that you came here. You want to learn how to perform Reiki healing. So, we mentioned Chi earlier, that energy that's inside us and all around us. When it comes to the body, your Chi travels along paths inside it called Meridians. These Meridians help ensure the flow of Chi where it needs to go in your body. Think of them as 'Chi Superhighways'.

Now, when the Chi is blocked or otherwise imbalanced (too much Chi here, too little Chi there) then the problems start and the longer that it's harmony is imbalanced the worse it can get. Resulting in something as innocuous as a bad mood on a particular day and up to more serious conditions like bipolar disorder or even heart problems.

This is serious stuff, folks. Why do you think a culture as old as China still utilizes Meridians in acupuncture and other treatments?

People like to scoff but despite the progress of current medical science, these ancient concepts are obviously doing something for millions around the world that's actually working.

So, we've established that Chi needs to flow properly and that Meridians are the roads that it utilizes in your body, next we should logically talk about Meridians. These are going to seem complicated at first as you'll need to memorize, over time, the circuitous paths that they take through the body. As a homework assignment after you read the rest of this chapter, get a piece of poster board at the store, then do a Google search and copy diagrams of the Meridians so that you can make a collage of their locations. Hang it up in the house somewhere where you'll see it often. You'll be going through exercises in the following chapter that will teach you exactly what paths the meridians take but creating a creative visual aid can help immensely as you begin your path as a Reiki Healer.

If you're ready, let's discuss Meridians. Applying this knowledge will take a little practice, but once you understand the pathways that the Chi energy takes through your body, then you'll understand how to better manipulate these energies within the framework of Reiki.

If you're ready, let's continue to the individual healings of the 12 Meridians.

THE 12 MAJOR MERIDIANS

While the Meridians are identified by particular parts of the body, that doesn't mean that they only govern that part of the body. It's a little more complicated than that but we're going to cut through the haze for you, cut it down into bite-sized chunks, and ensure that you get the understanding that you require. After all, we aren't writing an encyclopedia entry here, our job is to give you just what you need to get started and get practicing.

1. **Kidneys**- Producing bone and marrow through a chemical called EPO, kidneys also store sexual energy and regulate the development of sexual organs. You'll notice that we mention Asthma and Tinnitus as well, this is because these issues can be due to deficient kidney Chi. Be sure to take care of this meridian.

Location: Starting from the sole of your foot, this Meridian then travels up the inside of your leg, then to your abdomen and terminating just below the clavicle.

Physical effects:

- Tinnitus
- Asthma
- Backache
- Urinary issues

Emotional effects: This Meridian controls your force of will. A blockage or imbalance in this Meridian can cause a feeling that you're lacking control in life, unable to effect change no matter how hard you try.

2. **Spleen**- The Spleen performs a number of important functions. Regulating your blood flow, for one, and also regulating your digestion. As it's an important part in the transport of nutrients and their accompanying Chi, it also regulates your muscle density.

Location: This Meridian starts just outside of your big toe, coming up the inside of your leg to your thigh. It continues to your abdomen and up further, passing the outside of the nipple to your second rib, where it starts down again and terminates at the 6th intercostal space (6th space in your ribs, counting down from your head)

Physical effects:

- Abdominal issues (constipation, diarrhea, bloated feelings)
- Poor muscle density
- Prolapsed internal organs
- Chronic fatigue

Emotional Effects: Blockage or imbalance in this Meridian can cause you to feel mentally slow or absent-minded.

3. **Liver**- The Liver governs the menstruation and the female

reproductive cycle. It's also responsible for your tendons and ligaments. Most importantly, this organ is among the most important for storing and circulating Chi throughout your body.

Location: Starting inside your large toe (underneath the nail), this Meridian runs up the inner leg, up to your thigh, and then travels to the outside of your abdomen on the way to its terminus, which is your sternum.

Physical effects:

- Stiff joints
- Menstrual issues
- Vertigo
- Jaundice
- Blurry vision or dry eyes
- Headaches

Emotional Effects: Blockage of this Meridian can lead to a number of negative effects, such as anger, depression, and limited range of emotional expression due to an 'emotional lockdown'.

4. **Heart**- As the steward of your veins, arteries, and capillaries, the heart is immeasurably important to your physical health. It's also quite important to your mental health, as well. See below.

Location: This Meridian is a bit less complex to trace than the others. It starts in your arm pit, travelling down your inner arm and terminating at the fingernail on your pinky (smallest) finger.

Physical effects:

- Insomnia
- Dizziness
- Chest Pains
- Shallow breathing
- Cold sweats and hot flashes
- Bipolar disorder (from prolonged blockage or imbalance)
- Tachycardia/Heart Palpitations

Emotional Effects: This Meridian relates to your happiness. As such, it can cause a number of psychological issues if blocked, such as bipolar disorder, anxiety, depression, and obsessive-compulsive disorder. It also directly associates with an aspect of Chi called 'Shen', which is essentially our spirit and mental health... the presence that we exude. A number of issues can occur with imbalance, as you see, so be sure to perform healings upon this Meridian should you suspect that something is amiss.

5. **Lungs**- Your lungs regulate not only your respiration but also your intake of Chi energy.

Location: Starting at the first intercostal space between your ribs (the space between your first and second rib, starting underneath your head), this meridian goes up the shoulder and down the front of your arm, terminating at the fingernail of your thumb.

Physical effects:

- Problems with your sense of smell
- Upper body sweating and inflammation
- Coughing and congestion
- Skin conditions

Emotional Effects: A number of effects can occur when this Meridian is out of balance, such as depression, intolerance, false pride, contempt, or even as an inability to process grief.

6. **Pericardium**- The membrane that encloses your heart. Aside from the governance of its Meridian, the Pericardium holds importance as an energy center of the body that you can draw upon for healings. This is because the Pericardium not only protects the heart but it dissipates excess energy from the heart which you can draw into your palm to distribute to areas that need it.

Location: Beginning on the outside of the nipple, this Meridian travels from here up your shoulder and then down the front of your arm, terminating at the fingernail of your middle-finger.

Physical effects:

- Stomach issues
- Heart issues
- Chest pains

Emotional Effects: Imbalance or blockage in the Pericardium Meridian can cause issues with personal expression/communication with others, as well as paranoia, and phobias.

7. **Gall Bladder**- Storing and excreting excess bile, problems with this organ's Meridian can some serious health and emotional issues as listed below.

Location: This Meridian takes a long path through the body, starting at the outer corner of your eye, going inside your head and downward, and then down the front of your shoulder. From here it enters inside of your abdomen and then out again, travelling further down on the outer side of your leg where it terminates at your fourth toenail.

Physical effects:

- Yellowish tinge to the tongue or skin
- Liver pain
- Feeling bloated

Emotional Effects: Imbalance or blockage of the Gall Bladder Meridian can cause feelings of rage, excessive pride, and an overly judgmental attitude.

8. **Bladder** - Responsible for excreting liquid waste from the body.

Location: This Meridian starts at the inner corner of your eye, where it then goes over the top of your head, moving down your back and legs until it terminates at the toenail of your pinky (smallest toe).

Physical effects:

- Back Pain
- Stiffness in your shoulders and neck
- All diseases of the Urinary system
- Chronic headaches

Emotional Effects: Blockage or imbalance of the Bladder Meridian can cause issues with emotional expression, a 'hair-trigger' temper, restlessness, and extreme frustration.

9. Stomach- The stomach digests your daily meals and extracts Chi from them, distributing it to your spleen and intestines.

Location: This Meridian begins just under the center of your eye, going down the face to the very edge of your jaw, and then back up to your forehead. From here, it travels down to your throat, continuing to the front of your abdomen, down the front of your leg, terminating at the nail of your second toe.

Physical effects:

- Digestive issues

Emotional Effects: Effects that can occur from blockage or imbalance of this Meridian include feeling unaccepted, nervousness, constant worry, and an increased urge to criticize others.

10. **Small Intestine**- Distributing nutrients throughout the body, as well as Chi extracted from digested food, Blockage of

the Small intestines can result in one or a number of ailments listed below.

Location: This meridian starts at the fingernail of your pinky finger, going up along the back of your arm to your shoulder. It travels down your shoulder and then back up to the neck, moving finally to your ear.

Physical effects:

- Acne
- Neuralgia
- Abdominal pain
- Lymph node swelling
- Weakness in your legs
- Always feeling cold
- Stomach distention
- Nerve pain

Emotional Effects: Negative emotional impacts from blockage or imbalance in this Meridian can include feeling unappreciated, indecisiveness, nervousness, and constant feelings of discouragement.

11. **Large Intestine-** The large intestine removes water from waste matter, absorbing it and excreting the solids.

Location: This Meridian starts at the fingernail of your index finger. From here, it goes up your arm, behind your shoulder, and then up to your face, terminating at your nose.

Physical effects:

- All abdominal pains are connected with this Meridian.

Emotional Effects: Blockage or imbalance in this Meridian can result in an Inability to hold on or to let go of people in your life.

12. **Triple Warmer (your body's thermostat)**- This isn't actually an organ, rather it's a concept of Chinese medicine. You might call it your metabolism, but that's over-simplifying things. The Triple Warmer regulates body temperature, metabolism, and liquids. As such, virtually every imbalance that relates to an organ is going to relate to the Triple Warmer as well. The Triple Warmer, dissected, looks like this:

- *Upper Warmer-* Governs the upper part of your body, including your head, neck, heart, lungs, and your chest.
- *Middle Warmer-* The area between your navel and your chest, including the liver (special, see below), spleen, and the stomach
- *Lower Warmer-* Also governs the liver, your bladder, and the kidneys.

As you can see, this one is a bit more complicated at first but to keep it simple, be sure to include this in the healing of any Meridian, as it's always going to be part of an imbalance.

Location: This Meridian starts at the nail of your ring-finger, going up your forearm and continuing over the back of your shoulder. From here it continues around your ear and terminates at your eyebrow.

Physical effects:

- All

Emotional Effects: As the Triple Warmer covers all of the body, then consider any emotional dissonance to require a healing of the Triple Warmer as well as the associated other Meridians.

THE THREE EXTRAORDINARY MERIDIANS

Now that we've discussed the 12 Major Meridians, we need to tell you about the Extraordinary Meridians. While there are 8 of them, only 3 will be used in Reiki healing. These 3 act like spiritual batteries, storing Chi power that can be circulated through the body as needed. We won't go into too much detail on each at this time, as they're a little advanced but we wanted to include this information so that would have knowledge of these further Meridians to explore. The 3 Extraordinary Meridians are as follows:

1. **Ren Mai** -'The Conception Meridian'

Location: Beginning inside your mouth on the very tip of your tongue, this Meridian follows a path down the front of the body until it's terminus at your perineum.

Function: This Meridian governs all of your Yin Meridians.

2. **Du Mai** - 'The Governing Meridian'

Location: This Meridian begins at your coccyx, where it then travels up the spine until it terminates at a spot just behind your teeth.

Function: This Meridian governs all of your Yang Meridians. It's also responsible for protective/defensive aspects of your Chi.

3. **Dai Mai** - 'The Girdle Meridian'

Location: Running parallel with your kidneys and your navel, this Meridian is so named because it wraps around the body like a girdle.

Function: This Meridian governs your sense of balance.

YIN AND YANG MERIDIANS: SPLEEN AND STOMACH

- *Lungs and Large Intestine*
- *Liver and Gall Bladder*
- *Kidneys and Bladder*
- *Heart and Small Intestine*
- *Pericardium and Triple Warmer*

Above is the listing of Meridian pairings for the Yin and the Yang. Your Chi requires these forces to be balanced and your Meridians are paired in relation to each other and their aspects. With Reiki healings and acupuncture, when an imbalance occurs then the associated organ of the pair must be healed as well, for it's also out of harmony with its paired Meridian. Thus, if you're performing a Lungs Meridian healing, you'll also wish to perform a Large Intestine healing, in order to restore their harmony so that Chi may flow unimpeded. Sound complicated? Don't worry, we've got you covered, as you'll see in the exercises. You'll find it's not difficult, only new. Let's continue to the next chapter, 'Reiki Healing Exercises' and we'll show you.

4

REIKI SELF-HEALING EXERCISES

Finally, down to the nitty-gritty! We've given you a little bit of a foundation to get you ready for this moment. It's time to learn how to perform your first Reiki healings. These healings may be done just once for an ailment or, better yet, multiple times. Issues that took awhile to develop can take longer to address, so just keep in mind that sometimes you'll want to do many treatments to ensure proper healing.

Before we get started with exercises, we should take a moment to advise you in regards to the importance of proper breathing. Proper breathing techniques can help you with a number of things, including dealing with pain, narrowing your focus when you need to be sharp, and relaxing enough to reach a proper meditative state. Is it complicated? Nope, or at least, it doesn't have to be. There are advanced techniques, of course, that can take quite a bit of time to learn. All you need to get started, however, is a simple exercise that we'll detail for you now.

Learn it, practice it, know it. It's primitive but it will get you where you need to go!

So, if you're ready, let's outline the steps for your first breathing exercise.

Breathing exercise

1. *Sit somewhere comfortable for practice. This way you don't have any distractions. Once you're used to measured breathing then it becomes second nature, indeed, in times of stress you might find yourself automatically employing breathing techniques that you've mastered. Once you're comfortable let's move on.*
2. *Inhale slowly for a count of four.*
3. *Hold the breath slowly for a count of 4.*
4. *Exhale slowly for a count of 4.*

That's it! Simple, but effective. You can try alternating your counts, for instance, inhaling for 4, holding for 4, exhaling for 3 to see how it makes you feel. Different combinations can produce different results.

Experiment with them to see what gets you feeling healthiest and most focused. It seems a simple tool at a glance but you might be surprised at the applications that you'll find.

Now that you know how to breathe properly, we're going to start you off with the Triple-Warmer healing, as this Meridian will need to be healed in conjunction with any other Meridians that you're treating. Due to its nature (regulation of body temperature, bodily fluids, and metabolism) the Triple Warmer is almost always going to be imbalanced when there is an imbalance with the other Meridians.

Getting into the habit of doing this can make your healings more efficient. One note, if you like, record yourself reading the steps of these healings and play it with a little music while you practice. Keep the music instrumental so that it's not distracting. This is a great way to learn a healing if you like a hands-free immersion rather than sitting and memorizing from the book. Typically Reiki healing will involve particular hand placements, and we'll go into those later, but this method allows you to perform Reiki and to commit the Meridians properly to memory.

Reiki Healing for each of the 12 Meridians

Triple Warmer

1. *Begin your breathing exercises, getting nice and relaxed.*
2. *Visualize your own Chi flaring around you as a bright white light surrounding you and inside of you. Try to get a feel for how it flows through your body. Do you feel the blockage that's present? If not, don't worry, this will come with time.*
3. *Place your hand, palm open and fingers spread slightly at the place over your Pericardium. As we mentioned before, it's the membrane enclosing your heart that drains excess energy, so we are going to take advantage of this. With your Chi energized through visualization, start pulling the excess*

energy into your palm. See it gathering as a ball of light, almost too bright to look into.

4. *We are going to now move the ball of light as we move our hand over the Meridian. It should be noted, many practitioners will just hold a hand over the head or chest and trace the Meridians through visualization. You can certainly do that if you like but it's good practice to practice tracing the Meridians at the beginning to learn them. You might find you actually prefer moving your hand, however, as it feels quite graceful. That said, Start by placing your open palm over the nail of the ring finger. Visualize the Meridian like an electrical cable made of its own white light. Move your hand with the ball of light and see it crackling with white Chi energy as you bring it up your arm to your shoulder, moving it over and behind your shoulder slowly as you bring it up to the top of your ear and stop at your eyebrow. See the ball of light getting smaller as it transfers the energy, finally disappearing at the terminus of the Meridian. You may notice warmth or tingling when you do this, don't worry, this happens sometimes as you become more advanced and it's a good thing.*

5. *Next, we must consider the Yin and the Yang relationship for this Meridian. The Triple Warmer is considered to be the Yang aspect of a pairing with its Yin component, the Pericardium. To ensure the balance, take more energy from your Pericardium to make another ball of Chi light and move your palm over the Pericardium meridian. This movement will be very close to the opposite of the Triple Warmer meridian. Move your open palm to be just over the outside of*

your nipple. Move your hand slowly up to the shoulder and then down your arm, stopping at the nail of the Middle finger. As before, see the ball of light slowly diminishing as it feeds the Meridian, charging it and destroying imbalance and blockages.

6. Move your palm over the Meridian patterns that you just traced in this healing, focusing to see if you still feel any blockage or imbalance, or if they feel energized now to you. It may take practice to develop the sensitivity to this so be patient. Some people are lucky enough to be able to do this naturally but most people will need a little practice. Don't worry if you're one of the latter because you'll develop the sensitivity soon enough.
7. If you sense no blockage or if you're still learning your sensitivity and not sure, then relax your breathing and consider your first healing done. Do you feel differently after this? Invest in a notebook or a blank book to journal your healings and progress, it's a good way to learn and to document your steps along the Reiki path.

Next, we are going to go over a healing for the kidneys.

Kidneys

1. *Begin your breathing exercises, reaching the inner calm where you're ready to undertake this working.*
2. *Visualize your own Chi flaring around and inside you as your awareness expands from your measured breaths.*
3. *Place your hand , palm open and fingers spread slightly, over*

your Pericardium. Draw forth the Chi energy into your palm, a white ball of healing light.

4. Move your palm, the ball of light travelling with it, through the path of the Kidney Meridian. You'll start at the sole of your foot, moving the light up the inside of your leg. Bring it up further still to your abdomen and higher still, to the clavicle bone. See the line of the Meridian as clearly as you can in your mind, now crackling with the healing energy that you collected from the Pericardium.

5. The kidneys possess a Yin aspect and the Yang of the kidneys is the Bladder. Draw another ball of light from your Pericardium and let's empower the Bladder Meridian. Move your palm and Chi sphere up to your face, to the inner corner of your eye. moving it up and over the top of your head and then down your back. Continue down your leg until you reach the foot and the ball dwindles to nothing at the nail of your smallest toe. As before, visualize the Meridian line as you commit it to memory through practice. See it winding through its path, filling with power as you send healing energy and purge blockage and imbalance.

6. Draw another healing sphere of Chi from your Pericardium and perform the Triple Warmer Healing to ensure that the organs you've healed and the body's regulator are all in harmony.

7. Trace the associated Meridians to feel for blockage. Feeling anything yet? Don't worry, keep practicing.

8. If you sense no blockage or are still learning your Meridians, feel free to consider this healing practice complete.

Practice, practice, practice!

Let's continue now to learn a healing for the Spleen.

Spleen

1. *Begin your breathing exercises, as previously.*
2. *As your consciousness expands, visualize your Chi, blazing brightly.*
3. *Place your hand, palm open and fingers slightly spread, over your Pericardium. Take the excess energy coming from the Pericardium into your hand, forming it into a ball of light.*
4. *Move your palm and Chi light-sphere down to your foot, to the outer edge of your big toe. Move it from here slowly up your leg and further up, to the thigh. Move it higher still, up the abdomen and bring it up to the outside of your nipple until you get to your second rib. Move it down again to the terminus. the 6th intercostal space of the ribs (the intercostal space is the space between your ribs). As with the previous healings, see the Meridian lines as you're tracing them. Watch them filling with the energy as the sphere slowly diminishes.*
5. *The Spleen is considered to be the Yin in it's pairing with the Yang of the Stomach. That said, let's balance the Yin and the Yang to ensure these organs function in harmony. Draw an energy sphere of Chi from your Pericardium again and move your hand up to your face, holding it just over the center of your eye. Don't worry, this light is very good for you. Begin moving it down your face to the edge of your jaw, then up to your forehead. Move your palm of light slowly and to your abdomen, where you'll take it down the front of your leg to*

your foot and the Meridian's terminus, your second toenail. Visualize the stomach Meridian shining brightly now, free from blockage and imbalance and complimenting it's other half of the Yin and the Yang, the Spleen.
6. Perform the Triple Warmer healing to ensure that we are being thorough.
7. Now that we've performed the healing, trace the Meridians with your palm again, both for practice and to see if you can feel them flowing with unimpeded Chi.
8. If you sense no blockage, consider the healing a success.

Let's move on to our next candidate, the Liver.

Liver

1. Begin your breathing exercises so that you're in the proper mindset.
2. Begin visualization of the Chi energy around you, the same energy that pervades you and everything in the universe. See it as a bright light surrounding and filling you.
3. Place your hand, palm open and fingers slightly outstretched, over the Pericardium. Draw the needed energy into an orb so that it's ready to be redistributed.
4. Move your hand with the healing Chi down to your foot. Starting at your big toe (visualize the line starting under the nail), trace your open palm up your inner leg and bring it up. Move it further up along the outside of your abdomen, watching as it feeds the Liver Meridian with white light crackling like electricity. Continue up to the sternum and you've completed the circuit. See the entire Meridian glowing

clean and bright with the energy that you've placed there and commit as much of it as you can to memory. Soon you'll know it like the back of your hand.

5. The Liver is considered to be the Yin aspect of its Yin/Yang pairing with the Gall Bladder. Move your and back to your Pericardium and draw forth more Chi. Feel it as a warmth in your hand and hear it crackling. We'll need a lot of energy, as this Meridian takes a long path through the body. Move your hand to the outer corner of your eye. Let the orb loose and see it going inside your head and downward towards the front of your shoulder. Catch it with your palm and bring it slowly down your abdomen, letting it loose again to go inside, as you move your palm downwards. See the orb coming back into your hand, smaller now as it expends its energies. Next, you'll move it down the outer side of your leg and take it gently to its terminus, the nail of your fourth toe. This one is a little more complicated but you'll learn it. Towards this end, try to see it glowing brightly in your mind's eye, filled with the energy that you fed into it. Your Gall Bladder and Liver Meridians are now working, once again, in youthful harmony.

6. Perform the Triple Warmer healing to rule out any imbalances that may have been caused by the Liver and Gall Bladder Meridians when they were in disharmony.

7. Trace the Meridians that we've just worked with via your open palm. See if you can feel the harmonies of the Meridians that you've just worked so intimately with.

8. If you sense no blockage, let's move on.

Heart

1. *Begin with your breathing exercises to get centered.*
2. *Open your perception and see your Chi power, burning brightly.*
3. *Place your hand over the Pericardium, with your palm open and your fingers spread slightly. Draw upon the excess Chi that your body is shedding and shape it into an orb. Take a moment to enjoy the wonder of its brilliance. Like a boxful of puppies or kittens, a baby's smile, ice cream on a hot summers day...this is the stuff of life.*
4. *Move the Chi energy in your open hand to your armpit. Now move it slowly down your inner-arm and take it gently you the nail of your smallest finger. Visualize the Meridian glowing fiercely from the energy you just requisitioned for it. Commit it to memory and let's continue to balance it's counterpart.*
5. *The Heart Meridian is the Yin of its Yin and Yang pairing with the Small Intestine. To heal the Small Intestine and restore full harmony to the twain, move your hand to your Pericardium, palm open and fingers spread slightly, and draw fresh energy into it and shape it as an orb in your mind. Move your hand to the opposite hand, holding it over the fingernail of your smallest finger. Move it upwards, over the back of your arm to your shoulder, the orb of Chi light becoming smaller as you progress. Bring it down from your shoulder and then back up to the throat. From here, bring tiny orb up to your ear where the last of the energy you collected will be absorbed in the Meridian. Note the Meridian,*

now free of blockage and empowered, blazing with light, and commit what you can to memory.
6. Perform the Triple Warmer to ensure thoroughness of this Health-working.
7. Trace all of the Meridians that we've worked with on this healing to see what the energies feel like to you. Do you still feel a blockage or do they feel like running-rivers of energy?
8. If you sense no blockage, let's continue.

Lungs

1. Start your breathing exercises in preparation for manipulation of your Chi.
2. See your Chi, around and within you, shining brighter than any searchlight.
3. Place your hand, palm open and fingers slightly spread, over your Pericardium so that we may collect the excess Chi energy. Draw it into your hand, a blazing sphere of healing light.
4. Move your hand upwards towards the top of your ribcage, stopping at the beginning of the Meridian. This will be the first intercostal space or, simply put, the first space between your first two ribs. Slowly move the Chi-light up your shoulder and let it move down the front of your arm, the ball decreasing in size as the energy flows into the Meridian. Continue down the front of your arm until you reach your thumbnail where the tiny orb will at last deplete it's energy. Take a moment to enjoy the sight of this Meridian, brightly

flaring and free of blockage before we continue to its Yin and Yang counterpart.

5. *The Lungs are considered the Yin i the Yin and Yang pairing that exists with its counterpart, the Large Intestine. Let's move our open-palmed hand back to the Pericardium and once more collect healing Chi energy. Gather up your sphere of white light and bring it with your hand down to the fingernail of your index finger. From here, bring it up your arm to the back of your shoulder, and as the sphere of light dwindles, bring it up furhter to your face and it's terminus, your nostrils.*

6. *Perform the Triple Warmer healing to ensure that this is also in balance and to ensure efficacy of this working.*

7. *Trace the Meridians with your hand to see what you feel. By now it's likely that you're developing sensitivity to these energies. Good job. Soon you'll be ready for other techniques as well.*

8. *If you sense no blockage, let's move on and don't forget, some healings may take multiple sessions so don't be afraid to perform this or other healings multiple times in a week.*

Now we'll move on to our friend, that 'electric company' of spare Chi, the Pericardium.

Pericardium

1. *Begin your breathing exercises, as always. Don't neglect proper breathing, it's much easier to enter the mental state needed for these workings.*

2. *See your Chi in all its glory, blazing around and filling you. We are ready to go..*
3. *Place your hand, palm open and fingers slightly spread, over your pericardium. As we are doing a healing for the Pericardium, as you attempt to draw energy, meantally pull at some of the Chi that's surrounding you as well. You're one with the Universe, so drawing this energy is simply borrowing from yourself. It replenishes.*
4. *Move your open hand and hold it over the space just outside of your nipple, taking it slowly up your shoulder and then down the front of your arm. See the ball of light diminishing and feel any blockages exploding in the healing light of your Chi and you move the dwindling orb to this Meridian's terminus, the fingernail of your middle finger. Take a moment to admire this Meridian of light that serves the body as a pathway for your Chi. Soon you'll know this pathway by heart.*
5. *As we are familiar with the Yin Yang pairing already (the Pericardium pairs with the Triple Warmer), perform the Triple Warmer Healing to continue.*
6. *Traces the Meridians of both the Pericardium and the Triple warmer to see what you feel. Do they feel blocked still? Harmonious? They should feel healthy and restored after the working.*
7. *If you sense no blockage, we may continue to the Gall Bladder.*

Gall Bladder

1. *Begin your breathing exercises to prepare.*
2. *With each time you practice, it becomes easier and easier to see the Chi around you. Take a moment to congratulate yourself for your patience and perseverance. Bask in your Chi a moment and let's continue.*
3. *Place your hand, palm open and fingers slightly spread, over your Pericardium. Draw the excess Chi and feel it filling your hand with warmth and healing power.*
4. *We described the healing Meridian-path of the Gall bladder when we discussed the Liver, however, as it's one of the more complicated Meridians to memorize, we'll list it again for you.*
5. *"Move your hand to the outer corner of your eye. Let the orb loose and see it going inside your head and downward towards the front of your shoulder. Catch it with your palm and bring it slowly down your abdomen, letting it loose again to go inside, as you move your palm downwards. See the orb coming back into your hand, smaller now as it expends its energies. Next, you'll move it down the outer side of your leg and take it gently to its terminus, the nail of your fourth toe." Move your hand over your Pericardium and collect more healing light from your Chi. Direct the orb with your hand over the Liver Meridian from earlier in this chapter.*
6. *Perform the Triple Warmer healing.*
7. *Trace the associated Meridians to feel for blockage or imbalance.*
8. *If you're satisfied with what you sense from the Meridians, it's time to move on.*

Bladder

1. *Begin your breathing exercises to get properly relaxed.*
2. *Visualize your Chi, powerful and blazing around and within you, ready for this working.*
3. *Place your hand, palm open and fingers slightly spread, over your Pericardium. Collect the excess Chi energy into your palm in a ball of white light.*
4. *Move your hand up to your face to the inner corner of your eye, where it then goes over the top of your head. As the Chi-light slowly diminishes while empowering the Meridian, move it down your back and legs until it the Meridian terminates at the toenail of your pinky (smallest toe) and fully absorbs the Chi sphere.*
5. *As we learned from a previous healing in this chapter, the Bladder is the Yang of the Yin and Yang coupling it has with the Kidneys. Collect more energy from your Pericardium and perform step 4 from the Kidneys healing to empower the Kidney Meridian for balance.*
6. *Perform the Triple Warmer healing to ensure balance.*
7. *Check the Meridians from this healing with your hand and your growing sense for energies.*
8. *If you sense no blockage, we can move on to our next healing.*

Stomach

1. *Begin your breathing exercises to get centered.*
2. *Once centered, open your awareness to see your Chi energy around you and inside you. We are ready to continue.*

3. *Place your hand, palm open and fingers spread lightly, over your pericardium. Pull the excess Chi energy from it and let it form into a ball of blazing light.*
4. *Move your hand up to your face, just under the center of your eye. Move the Chi-sphere in your hand down to the edge of your jaw, then up to your forehead. From here, move your hand down your throat slowly as the energy from the sphere enters the Stomach Meridian. Continue down the front of your abdomen, down the front of your leg until you arrive at its terminus, your second toe.*
5. *The Stomach Meridian is the Yang of the Yin and Yang pairing it enjoys with it's Yin, your Spleen. Draw energy once more from your Pericardium and heal the Spleen Meridian (only performing step 4 from the healing listed earlier in this chapter)*
6. *Perform the Triple Warmer Healing in order to ensure that the previous blockage has caused no imbalance.*
7. *Trace the Meridians associated with this healing to ensure that the flow of Chi through these Meridians is healthy and unblocked.*
8. *If you sense no blockage, consider the healing a success.*

Don't worry, we only have two more to go. We hope that you've taken our advice from earlier and created a journal for your progress. This is often the best way to get a good idea how you're advancing and also to keep track of how often that you're practicing. Reiki is a rewarding path for a long and healthy life. That said, without further ado, Let's move to the first of the last two healings in this chapter, your Small Intestine.

Small Intestine

1. *Begin your breathing exercises and clear your mind so that you'll be receptive to your Chi,*
2. *Visualize your own Chi, enveloping you from head to toe in brightest of lights, pure life and divine bliss.*
3. *Place your hand, palm open and fingers slightly spread, over your pericardium. Pull the excess Chi energy into your hand in a ball of blazing white.*
4. *Move your palm and Chi sphere to your opposite hand, bringing the light to the start of the Small Intestine Meridian, your pinky (smallest) finger. Move the sphere up the Meridian, which is up the back of your arm to your shoulder. See the orb diminishing in size as you continue up to the neck and to the Meridian terminus at your ear. See the Meridian crackling with energy. From practice with the previous Healings it's likely quite familiar to you by now, almost an old friend. Let's continue.*
5. *The Small Intestine is the Yang component of its pairing with the Yin Heart. Reaching over to your Pericardium, gather more excess Chi light into an orb and use that orb to heal the Meridian for your Heart to balance the two Meridians. Employ only step 4 from the Heart Meridian Healing.*
6. *Perform the Triple Warmer healing in order to ensure balance.*
7. *Check the Meridians with you hand, open palm and fingers*

slightly spread, tracing their pathways to feel their energies. Do they feel more balanced?
8. If you sense no blockage, we are ready to continue to the last of the healings from this chapter for you to practice.
Good job.

Large Intestine

1. Begin your breathing exercises so that you may be receptive to your Chi energies.
2. Visualize your Chi, bright and powerful from your practice and previous healings.
3. Place your hand , palm open and fingers slightly spread, over the Pericardium. Draw up the energy that we'll need into a healing orb and let's continue.
4. Move your hand and healing Chi to your opposite hand, targeting the fingernail of your index finger. Move the healing sphere up your arm, watching as it gets smaller as it expends energy in destroying blockage and empowering this Meridian. Continue moving the healing light up and behind your shoulder and then up to your face, depleting the orb as it terminates at your nostrils.
5. The Large Intestine is the Yang to its Yin of your Lungs. Move your hand to your Pericardium and draw another Chi healing sphere's worth of energy and then use it to trace and heal the Lungs Meridian. Heal the Meridian only, don't perform the full Lungs healing.
6. Perform the Triple Warmer healing in order to ensure proper

function now that the Large Intestine and Lung Meridians are again in harmony. i
7. *Use your sensitivity, becoming more honed with your practicing to check the integrity of the Meridians that you just healed.*

If you're happy with the results of this healing, then you're ready to move on.

This concludes our chapter on Reiki Self-Healing exercises. Next we are going to discuss the Three Pillars. a foundational Reiki working set that Mikao Usui developed both for use before healings or even as part of your daily routine. We're going to follow that with a Tradition-based Reiki healing where you'll learn the traditional hand-placements now that you've enough knowledge of Meridians to utilize them. This is where it all comes together.

5

THE THREE PILLARS AND REIKI HEALING FOR OTHERS

The Three Pillars of Reiki

Aside from the 5 Principles of Reiki, Usui taught the Three Pillars as a form of foundational practice for Reiki. These meditations should be performed before each session (some like to perform the Gassho meditation every morning) and the guidance portions will help to hone your intuition into something you can trust easily.

So, to begin, we'll tell you about each Pillar and then we'll provide information on how to observe the Pillars before you perform a Reiki Healing.

1. **Gassho** - Translating as 'Two hands coming together', Gassho is many things, among them a moment of cleansing followed by what amounts to a spiritual statement of intent. Lastly,

projecting the feeling of gratitude to the collective conscious for the healing that you're about to perform.

2. **Reiji-Ho** - Translating roughly as 'the indication of Reiki power', Reiji-Ho is essentially asking for your hands to be guided. This aids in your goal of becoming intuitive about what Meridians are out of balance with little to no effort.

3. **Chiryo** - Translated as 'Treatment', this part is all about action rather than meditation. HHaving performed Gassho and Reiji-Ho, the practitioner begins the laying of hands in places where it's required. At first, you'll be utilizing the standard order of hand arrangements as you learn the body placements but eventually, through Chiryo, you'll develop a sense for where to place them.

So how does one invoke these Pillars? Well, with Chiryo it's, as we said, simply practice. For the first two you'll access their energies in this fashion:

Gassho invocation

1. Find somewhere comfortable to sit (you can do this standing if you like, whatever you're most comfortable with).

2. Begin your breathing exercises to get in the proper frame of mind.

3. Close your eyes and bring your hands in front of you, closed in a 'prayer' position. Press your fingers close together and focus your attention to the tip of your middle fingers. Recite the 5 Principles of Reiki:

Just for today, do not be angry

Just for today, do not worry

Just for today, be grateful

Just for today, work hard

Just for today, be kind to others.

4. When you're finished, project your feelings of gratitude to the Universe, to the collective consciousness... and you're done.

Next we'll continue to the guidance portion of your pre-healing routine. Invocation of Reiji-Ho will help your intuition immensely and the effect is cumulative, as you'll soon see.

Reiji-Ho Invocation

The Reiji-Ho invocation is done in 3 small parts.

- **Part 1:** With your hands positioned as before when you performed Gassho, close your eyes and ask for the Reiki power to flow through you. Visualize energies of all colors coming from all directions into you, brightening your Chi like a star. You're now empowered for your healings.
- **Part 2:** Ask the Universe for the issue to be healed. Ask for their recovery on all, even the unexpected levels.
- **Part 3:** Ask the Universe and the Reiki power to guide your hands, bringing them where they're needed so that your patient may be healed wholly.

Now you may continue to Chiryo, where you practice your Reiki healing hand positions. In time, you won't have to do all of them, just the ones that are needed.

Let's continue now to your first Tradition-based Reiki healing. It will be much easier than you're expecting. Now that you know the Meridians, all you need for Reiki healing is the proper mindset, the Pillars, and your hard-earned knowledge of the Meridians.

Excited? Then let's continue.

TRADITION-BASED REIKI HEALING

In traditional Japanese Reiki, there are hand placements that are used for healing the Meridians. While typically you don't touch someone when you're doing the healing, you can lay hands upon them (with consent), hold your hands slightly over them in the correct locations, or place the persons own hands in the correct position with yours over them (good for the areas that are a little more private). Now that you've a working knowledge of the Meridians that you'll be working with you're ready for a tradition based healing. This requires no special ritual, so to speak. Basic placement over the affected areas and focus on the proper flowing of the Chi is all that's required. That said, a little explanation as you work can go a long way with your patient so that they understand exactly what you're doing. For future healings, simple hand placement in the correct areas combined with your knowledge of Meridians is all that's required. You can talk about your day with the patient as normal. Chi goes where it's meant to go by nature, all it needs sometimes is a little Reiki nudge.

Here are the steps that you can use to provide a tradition based Reiki healing for another person. Use these steps to learn the hand positions and soon you'll be ready to perform these healings on your own.

STEPS FOR REIKI HEALING

1. Have the recipient of the healing lay down flat on their back somewhere comfortable and easy to reach. When you become adept at Reiki, you might consider purchasing an old hospital bed or a massage table for your healings as these are the proper height for a Reiki session.

2. Place both open palms over your patient's pericardium. Let them know that it's function is expelling excess Chi and that you're going to be drawing that forth to redistribute throughout the body as needed. Let them know also that this treatment is completely non- invasive, involving only your knowledge of the flowing of Chi and the proper placement of your hands to nudge it along, as their body does the rest, and that the patient may feel free to have a nice chat with you as things continue without fear of disrupting the energies.

3. Place your hands in the **First Position**.

Location: Face, covering the eyes.

- *With the First position you'll be standing behind your patient, hands cupped slightly above their eyes. Don't touch, just hold the hands above (depending on your personal style and the patient's comfort level) Alternately, you may place the patients hands over their eyes and your own above them if that's more desirable to the one that you're healing.*

4. Hold your hands in place and feel the flow of Chi throughout the Meridians. See Chi flowing through them, destroying obstacles in its path so that the life energy flows freely along each Meridian, as it should.

5. Next we'll assume the **Second Position.**

Location: Top of the recipient's head.

- Bring your hands back slightly so that the inside of your wrists are touching at the top of the head and your hands are placed so there is one on each side, with your fingertips almost touching their ears.

6. Hold your hands in place and feel the energy flow of Chi, travelling through the body, empowered and stimulated to flow by your treatment. Keep your hands in place for as long as it feels necessary before moving on to the next position

7. Move your hands into the **Third Position.**

Location: The back of the Recipient's head.

- Ask your patient to lift their head slightly. For this position, touching is more convenient for you but this will, of course, be up to the recipient of this healing and their own personal comfort levels. If they're okay with touching, then hold both hands together underneath their head, supporting it comfortably. If they're not comfortable with touch, simply assume the same position with your hands and request they hold their head up for a moment until this part of the healing is complete.

8. With the Chi energy that you're holding in your hands the flow of Chi should be restored shortly and we may continue to the next position.

9. Now we'll place our hands in the **Fourth Position**.

Location: Covering Cheeks and chin and wrists almost touching the ears.

- The Fourth position involves cupping the patient's face from behind, thumbs should be level with the cheeks, fingertips touching or almost touching underneath the chin, and the heels of your hands almost touching their ears. This is another Position where the ability to touch is favorable but let's keep everything within the patients comfort zone.

10. Take a moment holding your hands in the Fourth position,

gently coaxing the Chi energy to go it's natural path. Feel the warmth as the current of Chi assumes it's natural flow.

11. You're ready to place your hands in the **Fifth Position**.

Location: Throat, and the Center of your Patient's chest.

- You'll place your right hand, slightly curled over the patient's neck. Place your left hand over the center of the chest, next to the Heart.

12. Leave your hands in this position as more of the excess Chi restores the proper flow of energy.

13. Moving beside your patient, place your hands in the **Sixth Position**.

Location: Center of chest/upper ribcage.

- Place your left hand over the left side of the ribcage, just under the breast level, and place your right hand over the right side of the ribcage.

14. Take a moment to focus on the energies flowing properly. Visualize the Meridians closest to this area as you empower them with your hand placement and the excess Chi. ,

15. You're ready now to place your hands in the **Seventh Position**.

Location: Your patient's Solar Plexus.

- Move your both of your hands down to the Solar Plexus/'Belly' area. This is just above the Navel.

16. Move your hands down further into the **Eight Position**.

Location: Your patient's Pelvic bones.

- Moving both hands down further still and pulling them apart slightly so that one hand is over each Pelvic bone, you've now assumed the Eighth Position.

17. Let the excess Chi drain further, coaxing the natural flow of Chi energy through the recipients body. When you feel that the energy is flowing at peak level, move on to the next position.

18. When you're ready, have the patient roll over onto their stomach. Now you may place your hands in the **Ninth Position**.

Location: Shoulder blades of your patient.

- Place your hands as before but this time on the shoulder blades, with your left hand over the left shoulder blade and your right hand over the right shoulder blade.

19. Feel the energy flow going from constricted to slightly widened, then from slightly widened to completely unobstructed. Once the Chi flow has been restored here from your hand placement we are ready to move on to the next.

20. Moving your hands down we are ready to stop them in the **Tenth Position**.

Location: The middle of your patient's back.

- For this position we are simply moving our hands slowly down until they're hovering over the central portion of the back.

21. Keeping your hands in place and visualizing the Meridian lines, observe as the Chi energy resumes a healthy flow.

22. Now we are ready to move the hands further down into the **Eleventh Position.**

Location: your patient's lower back.

- Moving further down, keeping your hands covering the left and right sides, move them over the lower back and stop, holding them in place.

23. Hold your hands in place until the energy flow of Chi feels healthy and productive.

24. Now we may move on to the **Twelfth Position**.

Location: Just above the tailbone.

- Move your hands down and hold over the area just above the tailbone (definitely no touching with permission.).

25. Hold your hands in place until you feel that any blockages have been erased and then we are ready to move on.

26. Move your hands down to the legs for the **Thirteenth Position**.

Location: Behind the knees and at the base of the ankles

- Place one hand over the space behind the knee and one hand over the lower ankle.

27. Hold your hands here and allow the flow of Chi to reassert itself while you visualize Chi energy flowing to the terminus points of the Meridians that terminate in your feet.

28. Move your hands to the final placements, the **Fourteenth Position**.

Location: The soles of your patient's feet.

- Reaching over or simply stepping in front of the patient, place your hands over but not touching the soles of their feet.

29. Take a moment again to feel the energy from the Meridians that terminate at this point.

30. The healing is complete. Ask your patient how they're feeling. Most will report feeling relaxed and refreshed, their Chi flowed restored to its proper, unobstructed flows.

Now you know the healings, the daily rites. What you do with them is up to you. In the next chapter we'll expand your knowledge, what you do with it, for good or ill, is up to you. Hopefully you won't go all 'dark Reiki' on us after all of this time, practice a little patience and you'll soon be a healer of merit. Keep what you've learned close, focus your morale, and above all: heal.

6

CHAKRA POINTS AND REIKI: ARE THEY COMPATIBLE?

Now that you've learned some basic Reiki healing we would like to introduce you to another system that can be used in conjunction with your current techniques to enhance and strengthen your results.

We're talking about Chakra Points.

So, what exactly are Chakra Points and are they really compatible with Reiki?

Chakra Points are a system of Hindu derivation that have a rather interesting scope. Based on writings called the 'Vedas', written between 1000 and 1500 years B.C., the actual word 'Chakra' translates out as 'wheel'. This is based on the belief that around you and inside of you is your life force, a spinning energy that turns the 7 Chakra-wheels inside of your body. If one of them is turning too fast or too slowly then it can lead to imbalances that must be addressed to be healthy both spiritually and physically.

My, my... this sounds a little familiar, no?

As you can see, these systems have quite a little bit in common. As such, incorporating Chakra points into your Reiki healing is a powerful way to enhance your current techniques, much like a blacksmith makes an alloy of two metals that turns out to be stronger than either one would be alone. Is hybridizing the system truly more efficient? Well, that's for you to decide.

We just provide you with the toolbox, what you decide to use and make from these tools is truly up to you.

Now that we've piqued your curiosity, we'd like to give you a brief introduction to Chakra points in this chapter, followed by another chapter with exercises so that you can practice incorporating the two systems to see if it's to your liking. Now, Chakras are basically 7 points of energy centers, which start at the base of your spine, climbing straight up to the top of your head. These Chakras are fed energy from channels in the body called 'Nadis'. Now, while Reiki has the Meridians, Nadis are similar in function but different in number. While there are 12 Meridians that you've memorized and used often by now, there are 72,000 Nadis.

Before you run screaming, no, we are not going to have you memorize them. You won't need to know them to use what we are about to teach you. Just your Reiki basics and the information about Chakra points that we are about to provide. So, without further ado:

CHAKRA POINTS - A BASIC PRIMER

Before we continue, it should be noted that we are going to simplify using Chakras within the framework of your Reiki healing. There are colors associated with the 7 Chakra points are actually the 7 colors of the rainbow and as this isn't only easier to remember but very, very practical for effective visuals in meditations, we are going to use the color names as the primary focus for your Chakra manipulation. 'Proper' names will be included within the description of each so that you're educated in the Sanskrit name and the most common names of the Chakras but for what we are doing, the color focus is just as effective and much easier to remember.

Remember, this is a guide for just starting out. Should you decide you wish to learn more about integrating Chakras and Reiki at a later date there is much reference material out there for you to explore. We are just here to get you started. Now, here are the 7 Chakras so that you may familiarize yourself with them before we begin practical applications in the next chapter.

The 7 Chakra Points and their Healing Applications

1. Red Chakra - Muladhara - Root Chakra

Muladhara in Sanskrit means 'Root' or 'Support', and as such is also known as the Root Chakra. Located at the base of the spine, This Red Chakra rules over your survival instincts. Fight or Flight, Self -Preservation.. It's the sovereign center of survival. As a results of this influence the Red Chakra also affects your reliance on material possessions to feel secure and accomplished at home. Sexually, it governs the urge for procreation in how it relates to you feeling secure in home and family.

Healing Associations

- Your lower back
- Your legs
- Your Hips
- Your coccyx
- Your sexual organs (if Male)

2. Orange Chakra - Svadhishthana -Sacral Chakra

Commonly known as the Sacral Chakra , the name of this Chakra in Sanskrit translates as 'Sweetness'. So what is its purpose and where is it? Located below the navel, the Orange Chakra is quite important for how we interface with life. The Orange Chakra governs how we process experiences in life and how we connect with others. Basically put, the health of this Chakra determines how we deal with triumph and tragedy and our very sense of self. From another emotional aspect, a healthy Orange Chakra allows us to utilize our inner strength for ourselves as well as others. Think of it as sort of a 'radio station of the self' in this aspect, if the Chakra is healthy then you and other can hear your music and announcements loud and proud, whereas a blockage makes the signal scratchy and hard to understand completely.

Healing Associations

- Your large intestine
- Your colon
- Your bladder
- Your sexual organs (if Female)

3. Yellow Chakra - Manipura - Solar Plexus Chakra

It's Sanskrit name translating as 'Lustrous Gem', the Yellow Chakra is located at your stomach. Where the Orange Chakra broadcasts your self-power like a radio station, the Yellow Chakra is the actual seat of said power. This Chakra is strongly tied to both your personal and professional life. To the personal portion of your life, it's your ability to understand yourself as you truly are. A blocked Yellow Chakra can lead to self-delusion, so deal with blockages quickly if you suspect there might be one here. From a personal and professional level, the Yellow Chakra determines how much you can communicate who you're to the world at large. It also reflects your personal abilities and skills. Meditations on this Chakra can be quite useful when acquiring new skills, so be sure pay attention to its health.

Healing Associations

- Your gall Bladder
- Your stomach
- Your kidneys
- Your liver
- Your pancreas

4. Green Chakra - Anahata - Heart Chakra

The translation in Sanskrit for the Green Chakra is fitting with it's 'Heart' appellation. It's name translates to 'Unhurt, Unstruck, and Unbeaten'. Located at the center of the chest, the Green Chakra governs how much we are able to love ourselves and others. As such, like the Orange Chakra, it can determine how we process our experience and the lessons of life. After all, questions such as 'Do I love myself' and 'Do others love me?' have a profound effect on whether we take a fall as a lesson or a punishment.

Healing Associations

- Your heart (of course)
- Your breasts
- Your lungs
- Your arms
- Your upper back

5. Blue Chakra - Vishuddha - Throat Chakra

In Sanskrit, 'Vishuddha' means 'Purification', and in governance aspects the Blue Chakra rules communication with the self and with others but in a very particularly way. Stay with us on this.

The Blue Chakra governs another very important aspect of life, *your creativity*.

The poets, writers, and artists of the world all require that the Blue Chakra remains unblocked, as it directly affects their ability to take a concept or abstraction and make it into something solid that the world may understand and enjoy. This Chakra is located at the base of your throat.

Healing Associations

- Your mouth
- Your ears
- Your thyroid
- Your larynx
- Your throat
- Your neck

6. Indigo Chakra – Ajna - Third Eye Chakra

While the common name, 'Third Eye Chakra' makes you think this is only for spiritual perception, the Sanskrit name is much more accurate when describing it's function. Translating as 'To perceive', the Indigo Chakra governs spiritual awareness, yes, but it also governs your ability to think logically, to perceive what is true in an unclouded fashion. The Indigo Chakra let's you take immediate problems or perceptions and then make a conscious decision to 'pull-back' and see things from a birds-eye perspective. Interpreting the bigger picture, if you'll. The Indigo Chakra is, of course, located just above the eyes in the center of the brow.

Healing Associations

- Your pineal gland
- Your lymph nodes
- Your brain

- Your sinuses
- Your eyes
- Your endocrine system

7. Violet Chakra - Sahasrara - Crown Chakra

'Thousandfold' is its name is Sanskrit, the Violet Charka is the seat of your Spiritual power. Located at the top of your head, this Chakra governs your connection with all things spiritual as well as your awareness of your connections with the universe. Foresight is also affected by the Violet Chakra, as knowing your place in the bigger picture gives you a stronger chance to accurately predict or know your future.

Healing Associations

- Your joints
- Your spine
- Your cervical vertebrae

Now that we've learned some basics about the Chakra system, let's continue to some exercises where we can incorporate this with your current Reiki skill set. The results from the pairing of two powerful systems can be extraordinary, as you're soon to find out. So, when you're ready, let's continue to our next chapter, 'Incorporating Chakra Points into Reiki Healing'.

7

INCORPORATING CHAKRA POINTS INTO REIKI HEALING

Now that you've had some grounding in the basics of Chakra points, it's time to put that information to some use. As an exercise, try each first the way that they're currently listed and then try adding Meridian practices that you've already learned. See what is most efficacious for you. Once we've completed these, we are going to continue to learn a little about another compatible energy called 'Kundalini', which can help to power up your healings and comes with the added bonus of increasing awareness. These are all just building blocks that we are stacking upon the Reiki foundation that you've already constructed. Extra tools in your toolbox. Let's continue with practical applications of the Chakra information that you've learned and we can go from there.

CHAKRA AND REIKI HEALING MEDITATIONS

Here is your list of meditations. Above all, be sure to practice what you learn here so that you can incorporate this information into your healing toolbox. This will be a little different from what you're used to. Let's begin.

RED CHAKRA AND REIKI HEALING MEDITATION: AFFECTED BODY PARTS:

- Your lower back
- Your legs
- Your Hips
- Your coccyx
- Your sexual organs (if Male)

1. *Find yourself someone comfortable to lay or to sit down. You might be here awhile so make sure it's a comfortable place, free of distractions. Draw power from your Pericardium when you're ready.*
2. *Place your hand, palm open, fingers spread just over your Red Chakra point (the base of your spine). It can be in front of you or behind you, but front is easier for comfort.*
3. *Close your eyes and begin your breathing exercises , as discussed in our Reiki meditation chapter.*
4. *Once you're relaxed, clear your mind and begin focusing on visualizing the Chi around your body. See it as a white light that surrounds you and pervades you.*

5. *Begin focusing this energy into your Red Chakra, which you'll see as a glowing red sphere. Say it's Sanskrit name, 'Muladhara'. As you say the name, see energy flowing in pulses, like flickering electricity. With each recitation, see the Chakra glowing a brighter and brighter red.*
6. *When the light is as its fullest, Look upon the Chi with your Red Chakra, see how they integrate in harmony. Contemplate this for a moment and we are ready to continue.*
7. *Begin reciting 'Health to my _____' for each associated body part. Example: 'Health to my lower back', 'Health to my legs'.*
8. *With each recitation, see the Chi energy flowing from you into the Chakra, which in turn brightens and sends energy to the body part on which you're focused.*
9. *When you've completed all of the body parts, slow your breathing and open your eyes.*

That's it. Your first Reiki and Chakra meditation. Practice this so that you may better familiarize yourself with the healing location associated with the Red Chakra. When you're comfortable, we may continue to the Orange Chakra.

ORANGE CHAKRA AND REIKI HEALING MEDITATION: AFFECTED BODY PARTS:

- Your large intestine
- Your colon
- Your bladder

- Your sexual organs (if Female)

1. *Go back to your comfortable spot or find yourself a new one. Note, Nature is good for this too, as long as you've a pretty place where you won't be disturbed. Feel free to make a dedicated place or to mix it up a little, whatever makes you most comfortable. Draw power from your Pericardium when you're ready.*
2. *Place your hand, palm open and fingers spread over the spot just below your navel. This is the location of your Orange Chakra.*
3. *Close your eyes and begin your breathing, as we did in the previous exercise.*
4. *Once relaxed, visualize your Chi burning brightly around you. Focus this energy to your hand.*
5. *Now we'll being focusing energy into your Orange Chakra, which you'll see as a glowing orange sphere. Begin repetitions of its Sanskrit name, 'Svadhishthana', and with each repetition see the Chi flowing from your hand into the Orange Chakra. which responds with blazes of orange fire until it's burning brightly.*
6. *Now that your Chi and your orange Chakra are both blazing and in harmony, take a moment of contemplation to see if any insights come on how these energies play together. It's important always to pause for contemplation as there are always new things to learn about the interplays of these energies.*
7. *Begin reciting as before, 'Health to my _____' for each associated body part.*

8. *See the Chi energy becoming Orange Chakra energy and direct that energy to each body part. Visualize them as best you can. In very powerful meditations, sometimes you'll feel a tingling or a warmth. Don't worry, this is normal.*
9. *When you're done all of the associated body parts, relax your breathing and open your eyes.*

Remember, practice makes perfect, and learning the Chakra associations with healing is our goal, so memorize but above all, practice these meditations.

YELLOW CHAKRA AND REIKI HEALING MEDITATION: AFFECTED BODY PARTS:

- Your gall Bladder
- Your stomach
- Your kidneys
- Your liver
- Your pancreas

1. *Find your favorite meditation spot and get comfortable. Feel free to add music to your meditations if you like, sometimes it helps for deeper and fuller meditations. Just nothing too distracting, we want the focus to be within and not without.*
2. *Place your hand, palm open and fingers spread over your Yellow Chakra, which is conveniently located at your stomach.*
3. *Close your eyes and begin the measured breathing portion of*

your meditations. Be sure to get good and relaxed for the best results, we don't want any distractions that come with a stressed and agitated mind.

4. *Let your awareness spread slowly from your center until it encompasses a few feet outside of the body. See your Chi, white light blazing and mysterious, at one with yourself and yet at one with the entire universe.*
5. *Properly humbled and yet also empowered, let's send some of this energy into the Yellow Chakra. See it as a glowing yellow sphere, like a perfect orb of clear Citrine filled with its own inner light. Begin repeating it's Sanskrit name, 'Manipura'. With each repetition see the white Chi light pouring into the sphere which is filling with golden light, as if with water. Once it's full, see it shining brightly and clear as glass.*
6. *Take a moment to contemplate the beauty of this interplay of energies. Ponder that the Yellow Chakra is the Chi and the Chi is the Chakra. It's a reflection of oneness with the self and the Chi energy of the Universe around you.*
7. *Recite, 'Health to my _____' for each associated body part.*
8. *As recite this, see light coming from your Yellow Chakra as if it were focused by a magnifying glass, like the 'water' of Chi power that you filled it with has enabled the Chakra a heightened focus. Feel a healing warmth as it touches each body part.*
9. *Once you've completed this, relax your breathing and open your eyes. You're done.*

Work, sleep, rinse and repeat. You'll find that you learn these meditations quite quickly, just be sure to make time on your schedule or better yet, practice one daily before work.

GREEN CHAKRA AND REIKI HEALING MEDITATION: AFFECTED BODY PARTS:

- Your heart
- Your breasts
- Your lungs
- Your arms
- Your upper back

1. *Get nestled in your meditation cove, comfortable and ready for this working.*
2. *Place your hand, palm open and fingers spread over your Green Chakra, which is located in your central chest area.*
3. *Close your eyes and relax. Begin your breathing exercises.*
4. *Open your awareness and see the Chi flowing around in and in you. Bask for a moment in the energy of the life of all things in the Universe.*
5. *Collect the energy around you and focus it into your hand as you visualize the green Chakra orb inside you. Say it's name, 'Anahata', repeating it like a chant as your Chi flows into the Chakra which, in turn, then fills organically as if plants of energy were growing upward and twining together until they join as one bright and shining whole.*
6. *Observe your proper contemplations as always. Just as you relate to the world with different aspects, each Chakra relates*

with your Chi in its own fashion. Observe, learn, and listen to the silence for a truth or two. We are not in a hurry.
7. *Recite, 'Health to my _____' for each associated body part.*
8. *With each recitation, see your Chi empowering the Green Chakra which in turn reaches out vines of green energy, wrapping the focus of each recitation in healing warmth, suggesting growth and regeneration.*
9. *Once you've addressed each of the body parts we've listed for the Green Chakra, relax your breathing and open your eyes anew.*

Your Green Chakra is now empowered and the healing is in place. Take advantage and spend some time with someone dear, you'll find yourself better able to feel and communicate. Give it a try.

BLUE CHAKRA AND REIKI HEALING MEDITATION

Affected body parts:

- Your mouth
- Your ears
- Your thyroid
- Your larynx
- Your throat
- Your neck

1. *Find your meditation nook and sit down comfortably.*
2. *Place your hand, palm open and fingers spread over your*

Blue Chakra point. This one is located at the base of your throat.
3. *Close your eyes and begin your breathing exercises.*
4. *As you become more and more relaxes begin to see your Chi flowing around you. If it doesn't seem bright enough around you, feel free to pull from the Universe to brighten it. You're one with the Universe so you're only borrowing from yourself.*
5. *Visualize a bright blue sphere underneath your hand. Say the proper name of the Blue Chakra, 'Vishuddha', and begin repeating it as a chant. See your Chi energy encircling and filling the sphere with blue light, starting from the edges and circling slowly as it fills the empty center.*
6. *Observe the interplay of the energies now that both your Chi and your Blue Chakra are in focus. Do you notice anything special in how they interact? You might consider keeping an insight journal for those moments of enlightenment that you wish to keep.*
7. *Recite, 'Health to my _____' for each associated body part.*
8. *With each repetition of 'Vishuddha', see your Chi energy empowering the blue sphere and bathing the body part that you're focusing upon in sapphire light. Feel a tingle as if from a cool wind on each, as if each has become healthy and antiseptic.*
9. *Once each body part has been addressed, let your breathing relax and open your eyes.*

Don't forget to practice this often. You may find yourself especially creative after this exercise, do some writing, a little bit of art... take advantage.

INDIGO CHAKRA AND REIKI HEALING MEDITATION: AFFECTED BODY PARTS:

- Your pineal gland
- Your lymph nodes
- Your brain
- Your sinuses
- Your eyes
- Your endocrine system

1. *You know the drill. Get comfortable and receptive to some deep workings. Now we are going to learn a Reiki healing that inorporates the Indigo Chakra. Let's continue.*
2. *Place your hand, palm open and fingers spread over your Indigo Chakra, which is located on your forehead, just above and between your eyes.*
3. *Close your eyes and begin your breathing exercises. Make sure that you're quite relaxed before continueing.*
4. *Visualize an Indigo sphere just under your hand opening slightly, like a sleepy eye as your Chi fills your vision, all around you and more brilliant than you've seen it previously. Take a moment of contemplation of this. Development of the Indigo Chakra can make you more sensitive to energies.*
5. *Say the name of this Chakra, 'Ajna', and begin repeating it in a chant. See the light of your blazing Chi flowing from your*

hand into the eye. See the Indigo eye becoming a deeper shade of indigo with each Chi infusion, opening wider as well until you feel a deeper awareness flooding inside you.
6. *Definitely take a moment of contemplation this time. See the energies around and inside you. At this moment you're likely more spiritually perceptive then you've ever been before, so it's best to take advantage.*
7. *Recite, 'Health to my _____' for each associated body part.*
8. *With each recitation, see the Chi energy flowing from your hand and directing the eye to gaze upon the body part where you wish it to focus. See the gaze as an indigo searchlight and each body part becoming clearly sharper in perspective and healthier with each full gaze placed upon them.*
9. *Once each body part has been sent healing energies from your Chi empowering the Indigo Chakra, relax your breathing and open up your physical eyes.*

This working may produce odd dreams or the occasional intuitions. From the logic aspects of this Chakra you might also find yourself a little better organized. Don't worry, this is normal, enjoy.

VIOLET CHAKRA AND REIKI HEALING MEDITATION: AFFECTED BODY PARTS:

- Your joints
- Your spine
- Your cervical vertebrae

1. *Let's prepare by going to our meditation zone. Put on your favorite meditation music if you like and let's prepare to do a Reiki healing with the Violet Chakra.*
2. *Place your hand, palm open and fingers spread over your Violet Chakra point. This one is located at the top of your head.*
3. *Close your eyes, begin your breathing exercises, and get nice and relaxed.*
4. *Become aware of your Chi around you, surrounding you and flowing through your body through the Meridians and the Chakras.*
5. *See the Chakra at tthe top of your head, a violet sphere glowing fiercely. Address it by its name, ' Sahasrara' and begin repeating the name slowly. As you repeat the name, see your Chi energy flowing into the Violet sphere, filling it with a crackling fog of energy which coalesces slowly into a shining purple brilliance.*
6. *Enjoy your moment of contemplation and ponder how the Chi around and inside you interacts with the seat of your spiritual conscience.*
7. *Recite, 'Health to my _____' for each associated body part.*
8. *With each recitation, see the Violet sphere growing brighter and brighter, with the outlines of a face sometimes appearing within. Your face. See the sphere, directed by Chi and your spirit, directing violet energy to each part of the body that you wish to send rejuvenation and healing to.*
9. *Once you've finished with each body part for this Chakra, relax and open your eyes. You're done.*

This rounds off our sample healings to get you a little practice with using Reiki in conjunction with your Chakra points. As we've mentioned, practice, practice, practice. You'll be surprised at the benefits that can come from this understanding of the body's energies so keep up your studies and absorb this wisdom. You'll be happy that you did.

8

REIKI AND KUNDALINI: ARE THEY COMPATIBLE?

Around 500 to 1500 years B.C., a Hindu text called the Upanishads makes mention of a path of spiritual enlightenment known as Kundalini. The root of its Sanskrit name, 'kundalin', translates out to 'circular', which reflects the visualization of the energy. Kundalini energy is spiritual energy that resides at the base of your spine at the Red Chakra, coiled around the spine like a snake. As such, it's often referred to as 'The Serpent Power'.

Sound familiar? In Greek legend, there was a healing staff known as the Rod of Asclepius. The Caduceus, similar in design but with two snakes is the one you're probably more familiar with, however, due to its eminence as a symbol of healing adopted by Health organizations in North America.

It's interesting that such symbols of power are cross-cultural.

The Serpent power, said to rise up from the Red Chakra and

stretching up to the Purple Chakra when a spiritual awakening has been achieved (and this is a good time to remind you that Mikao Usui had a spiritual awakening), you might think that this energy has very little to do with Reiki, which is primarily a healing system. In actuality, there are quite a few areas where Kundalini practice can't only have relevance, but where it can strengthen particular healing efforts and give us yet another useful tool in the growing toolbox of aspiring Reiki Healers.

For arguments sake, here are a few points in which Reiki and Kundalini coincide:

- Reiki involves laying the hands upon certain points in order to balance Chi. Chakras, a system we discussed before is similar, where health is reliant on the distribution of 'Prana', or life-energy. Kundalini incorporates Chakras heavily in it's system.
- Reiki requires you to unblock the Meridians so that Chi may flow. For spiritual awakening, Kundalini requires Sushumna, the central channel, as well as a number of Chakras to be unblocked before it may rise.
- Both teach principles of letting go of hate, compassion, and gratitude.
- Both disciplines possess powerful methods of healing the body and mind

These are just a few, of course. What matters most for us is the healing aspect. Medical doctors don't turn down new gear just because they're unfamiliar with it, if it can enhance their ability to heal.

In the next chapter we are going to introduce some exercises that you can try in order to determine whether Kundalini has a place in your own style or Reiki or not. You should be warned. As Kundalini is also geared towards spiritual awakening, should you begin getting headaches or having odd dreams then don't worry, these are just a few of the signs that you might be in for a spiritual awakening. If this occurs, spend a little more time with your Chakra works and perhaps invest in a little Kundalini research to help push it along. After all, even though healing is our primary goal, a little enlightenment never hurts. Let's continue to the next chapter and begin our exercises.

9

USING REIKI IN CONJUNCTION WITH KUNDALINI

Now that we've given you a little foundation on Kundalini concepts and history it's time to incorporate a little training with a popular Kundalini medium. Mantras. Mantras are sacred words that are used for a number of reasons... protection, enlightenment, or in this case, healing.

We've gathered a collection of Mantras that you can incorporate into your Reiki Healing framework. Some of them will take a little practice but we are certain that you'll be pleased with the results. So what is the next step? Find a Mantra, pick any one that appeals to you personally or simply work through the list. If you've been keeping a progress and contemplation journal then be sure to note it as you go. You may be closer to a profound experience right now than you think so if you've got it, then keep the journal handy. Draw some excess Chi energy from your Pericardium and let's begin.

REIKI AND MANTRA INTEGRATION EXERCISES

1. Mantra: **' Chattar Chakkar Varti'**

This is a Mantra that you can use in conjunction with Reiki Healing for anxiety. Touch your hand your skin and feel the Reiki healing energy flowing inside of you as you chant this Mantra (or mouth it silently if you're in a more public place). See the healing energy empowering your Chi to grow brighter, as light branches from the Chi into the body to the Solar Plexus Chakra. In this way you've employed aspects of Chakra Points and the Kundalini in order to compliment the powerful Reiki healing energies. Your fear will soon be banished.

2. Mantra: **'Sa Re Sa Sa'**

This Mantra is may be used to remove negativity at the same time that it stimulates your creativity. You'll need a notebook and a pen and pencil handy (not required, necessarily, but useful for this exercise) This Mantrat associates with your Throat Chakra, so for this Reiki healing, tap your throat as you say each word of the chant and see the white light of your Chi brightening with each tap of your finger and your Throat Chakra brightening in its own blue glow. When the light of your Chi and your Throat Chakra will grow no brighter, stop tapping, and write down the first thing that comes to your mind. This will be your inspiration for a great writing or artwork, so be sure to store the notebook somewhere safe where you may consult these results as needed.

3. Mantra: **'Ra Ma Da Sa Sa Say Sohung'**

This Mantra strengthens the body and the mind, stimulating them from within as the white light of your Chi brightens and expands in harmony with this working. Best used in the morning (but you can do this any time that you wish), to use it, first place your hand, fingers spread, and touch your forehead. Focus on the repetition of the Mantra and with each repetition, see the light spreading from your forehead and down as it brightens your entire Chi. As the light goes down your body, visualize a coil of energy, your Kundalini, at the base of your spine slowly uncoiling as it rises to the Crown Chakra at the top of your head. Repeat until your Chi will grow no brighter and then go about your day confidently with your healing factors stimulated.

4. Mantra: **'Hum Dum Har Har'**

This is a very powerful Mantra that can focus healing in a number of ways. It translates roughly into 'We are everything, the universe, and the Creative Infinity.'. It promotes tranquility for deep and healing rest as well as stimulating the Crown, Third Eye, and Sacral Chakra points. This allows for a more focused healing. The healing areas associated with these Chakras are as follows:

Crown Chakra

- Migraines headaches, Bipolar disorder, Thyroid issues, lack of inspiration

Third Eye Chakra

- Eye pain, insomnia, chronic headaches, loss of interest in your future

Sacral Chakra

- Bladder, back pain, Ovarian cysts, kidney problems, lack of sex drive

As you can see, there are a number of issues that may be targeted. For this healing, hold your hand open, fingers spread, and move it slowly from the Crown Chakra, down to the Third Eye, and then down to the Sacral Chakra as you chant the Mantra. Visualize light spreading from your hand and your Chi energy growing brighter as each of the three Chakras ignites in it's particular color. Violet for the Crown Chakra, Indigo for your Third Eye Chakra, and Orange for your Sacral Chakra. As your Chi blazes, move your hand to the specific Chakra area that concerns what you would like to heal. See it's light glowing as well, your Chi a circle of bright light white with the Chakra's light in the center, working in harmony. When you feel focused and centered in these energies (and you'll know) then visualize the specific area of the body that you're working to heal. See energies from your Chi and Chakra striking the area like a warm, healing lightning. Once you can visualize this and feel it's warmth, bask in it until you feel ready and then relax your breathing and open your eyes.

5. Mantra: **'Wahe Guru'**

Translating roughly into 'The ecstasy of divine wisdom that

can't be described', this Mantra may be employed for lifting the spirit, strengthening the Chi, and increasing the speed at which you learn to manipulate energies. It's a Mantra of self-transformation and as such, can be one of the most healing Mantras of all. To use it, place your hand upon your face and see your Chi energy shaping brightly around you, forming an arrow pointing to the north that grows more sharply distinct with each repetition of the Mantra. Feel your mind sharpening in focus as well and think of your goal, your energies will be more aligned to the achievement of it.

6. Mantra: **'Ek ong kar sat nam siri wha hay guru'**

This Mantra is known as the 'Adi Shakti'. It translates roughly as 'In the ecstasy and bliss of Wisdom, the Creator and Creation are one'. It associates with the Solar Plexus Chakra and as such, using it with Reiki can help to focus an energy healing to the associated areas, such as the Gall Bladder, stomach, the liver, and the pancreas. To use this Mantra with a Reiki healing, hold your hand, palm open and fingers spread, over your Solar Plexus Chakra. Begin chanting the Mantra as you visualize rippling white light in your Chi with the Chakra Point glowing a brighter and brighter yellow in a solid sphere. Visualize the area that you wish to heal as well (google a picture of a healthy version of the organ that you wish to send healing energy to as an aid in your visualizations). Move your hand from the Solar Plexus Chakra to the afflicted area and see a synthesis of the White Chi and Yellow Chakra energy moving into the area.

Feel a rising heat in the area, not unpleasant, only soothing and continue the visualization and the chant for a few minutes until you feel the healing energy is well in place. Open your eyes and you're done.

7. Mantra: '**Har Har Har Har Gobinday**'

This is a healing Mantra for the Mind, specifically for the negative results that can occur with over-contemplation of a rocky past. While it's good to learn from the past, dwelling there can cause you to trip and falter on your path to a brighter future. Use this Mantra as needed to help in dispelling the negativity so that it no longer binds you from moving forward. It associates with the Sacral Chakra which, among other things, impacts the way that we interpret the various experiences of life, be they life-affirming such as the birth of a child or deeply wounding, such as the death of someone dear.

To use this in a Reiki healing, hold your hand, palm open and fingers spread, above the Sacral Chakra. This is just below the Navel. Visualize your Chi energy flaring around you as bright white light and your Sacral Chakra responding in kind with it's deep orange light. As you chant the Mantra, see an Hourglass inside the Chakra light, full of sand at the bottom. Let the white light of your Chi energy extend inside to force it over, so that new pasts may be built on the sands of the old. Feel the old oppression losing it's hold on you. Open your eyes, confident in the knowledge that the Past is no longer everything, but rather, the steps we took to get to the steps that we now take.

8. Mantra: '**Har**'

Translated as 'The Creative Infinity', this Mantra may be utilized in Reiki healing as a means of repairing the damaged inspiration. Are you having Writer's block or trouble with an Art concept that you're developing? This Mantra can help. One of the functions of the Throat Chakra, which this Mantra associates with, is the expression of Creativity. To break the dam and let the river flow, use the following steps. First, hold your fingers close to your throat. See your Chi energy flare up as you begin the chant. The white light surrounds you and you'll let it flow like water, down from the Crown Chakra at the top of your head, past the Third Eye Chakra between above and between the brows, and finally to the Throat Chakra which will flare a bright blue. Imagine that there is an impediment here, a tiny wall which is preventing the Chi from flowing downward to the Root Chakra. Now visualize the energy pushing through violently, breaking the blockage and travelling downward through your lower Chakras. The blockage destroyed, see the Chi power travel down, like in a completed electrical circuit, until it reaches the Root Chakra. Now it travels back up, igniting each of the 7 Chakras in their colors.

Red, Orange, Yellow, Green, Blue, Indigo, and Violet..

As the Chi energy travels back up, it also moves outside of the body at the same time, creating a nimbus of light with 7 Chakra gems at the center. Enjoy the brilliance and open your eyes, it's time to express your creativity.

9. Mantra: ' **Gobinde, Mukunde, Udare, Apare, Haring, Karing, Nirname, Akame**'

This Mantra translates as 'Sustainer, Liberator, Enlightener, Infinity, Destroyer, Creator, Unnamed, Without Desire'. Tied to the Heart Chakra, this Mantra can help the brain to function by lessening disharmonies. This can be used to ward off social anxiety, paranoia, false suspicions on your part, or the inability to interpret emotional responses due to disharmony of the heart and the mind. It can also be used in conjunction with your current medical regimen for irregularities of the heartbeat such as Tachycardia.

To use this Mantra with Reiki healing, hold your hand just over your Heart Chakra (your central chest) and visualize a green light growing forth organically to fill the sphere of energy of your Heart Chakra. Begin your chanting of the Mantra. See it as if the light is pulsing, in tune with your heartbeat and the individual words of the Mantra. Next, visualize your Chi energy pulsing as well, synchronized with your Heart Chakra.

If there is a particular area you wish to promote healing in, visualize it as each flash occurs. See the flashing going faster, out of synch with your heart now, until both lights of the Chi and the Heart Chakra are now a solid light and the visual of the area you wish to heal is solid, in the center of both. When you feel suffused with the healing warmth you may open your eyes, your energies are now aligned towards this healing.

10. Mantra: "**Om**"

'Om' is the sound that the Hindus believe was the first sound heard in the creation of the Universe. This Mantra can be used to heal blockages of the Throat Chakra and consequently, the areas associated with the Throat Chakra (neck, mouth, ears, the thyroid, and the Larynx). To use this Mantra with Reiki, hold your hand close to your throat, cupped, just below the chin. As you chant the Mantra, notice how it reverberates. See yourself surrounded by your Chi and pull back your vision to see the same energy surrounding you in everything. See the Throat Chakra flare up as your Chi brightens in tune with it. Continue chanting and visualize the blockage being broken or the part of the body you wish to heal glowing with a combination of both lights. Continue to pull out your view as you chant. Feel the Infinite around you before 'dropping back' to your body. Open your eyes, the working has been performed and may be repeated as needed.

11. Mantra: ' **Prana, Apana, Sushumna, Hari. Hari Har, Hari Har, Hari Har, Hari**'

'Prana' is the Hindu word for 'Life Energy', while 'Sushumna' is the 'Central Channel' through which your energies flow. Much like the Midians, actually, which is one of the reasons these systems work well together. This powerful Mantra may be used to speed up healing. To use it for a Reiki session, place your hand just in front of the center of your chest, not touching but almost touching your skin. Begin chanting the Mantra as you visualize your Chi energy moving up slowly from the base of your spine to the afflicted area.

See the area glowing with Chi light of it's own' in harmony with the Chi that surrounds your body as well as the Chi in the Universe around you. Continue the chant and the slow send of energy upwards until you feel the tingling warmth that lets you know that the energy is going where it needs to go. Now, you're done. Try this a few times a week to speed your bodie's natural healing.

12. Mantra: 'Ong Sohung'

Bearing a rough translation of 'I am the creative consciousness', this Mantra may be used in conjunction with Reiki for the healing of areas associated with the Heart Chakra (heart, breast, lungs, and upper back.). To use this, Hold your hand, palm open and fingers spread over your Heart Chakra.

Chant the Mantra in tune with the beat of your heart, one word per beat, as you visualize Chi energy flowing through your hand and filling your Heart Chakra with energy, creating a glowing green gem at the Chakra point. See the energy flowing from here to the afflicted area, infusing it with light and warmth. Do this until it seems that it can no longer contain energy and then relax your breathing and open your eyes.

13. Mantra: "Akal, Maha Kal"

With a grim translation of' Undying, Great death, this Mantra may be used with a Reiki healing to remove anxiety and fear. As we are relaxing the mind of anxiety, place your hand, palm open with fingers spread over your Solar Plexus Chakra. As you say the first sacred word, 'Akal', see the white light from your Chi flowing into your Solar Plexus Chakra and as you say the second part, 'Maha Kal' see the Chakra responding by igniting with orange fire.

Feel the fire chasing away your anxiety. Feel it burning up the fear. Repeat the Mantra and keep feeding Chi energy to empower it, until the fire of the Chi and Chakra energy has devoured all or enough of the fear and you can face things with a calm mind.

14. Mantra: ' **Ad Guray Nameh, Jugad Guray Nameh, Sat Guray Nameh, Siri Guru Devay Nameh**'

Roughly translated, 'I bow to the primal teacher who takes us to the divine inspirations, I bow to the elder wisdoms, I bow to the true and hidden wisdom.'. This powerful Mantra can be used as a preventative measure from toxic personalities or as a defense from chronic anxiety. To use this in a Reiki healing (though in this case, 'preventative healing'), hold your open palm, fingers spread over each Chakra point from Root to Crown.

Visualize your Chi blazing around you, a protective white sphere of light, and begin your chant. Visualize the Chakra energies extending on both sides as you empower each, forming a crystal lattice of all of their associated colors within the circle. It may take more than one chant of the Mantra to empower each Chakra but that's okay, just do it slowly and chant as many times as you need to create the protective sphere. Once you can see it in all its glory, open your eyes and go about your day in confidence.

15. Mantra: ' **Sat Narayan, Wha He Guru, Hari Narayan, Sat Nam**'

While there isn't a full translation available, Hari Narayan is essentially 'sustenance of creativity', as 'Narayan' represents the fluidity of shape that's possessed by water. This Kundalini

Mantra may be used in a Reiki healing to promote clarity of thought or to promote healing. To invoke this, place an open palm on each side of your headd, fingers lightly touching the skin. Begin chanting the Mantra and see your Chi energy entering your body through your head and flowing down to the spine.

When it reaches the spine, see your Kundalini energy uncoiling from the base of your spine like a serpent and stretching slowly up to your Crown Chakra. When the energy is fully extended, let bothyour Chi and your Serpent power become brighter and brighter until their brilliance is hard to look into. Feel peaceful and safe in this glow, balanced and at one with yourself and with the Universe. This Mantra is also very good when you've just suffered a shocking or traumatic experience and wish to balance yourself by balancing your energies.

Be sure to practice your Mantras. Paste reminders on the refrigerator or on post-it notes throughout your home or work desk. There are a number of ways that you can help to remind yourself, the number one method is going to be practice, practice, practice.

We hope that you've enjoyed this new addition to your toolbox. There are more Mantras out there for you to discover, should this chapter have piqued your interest. While Mantras may serve a wide variety of purposes we wanted to provide you with the ones that fit best with our healing framework. After all, this is 'Reiki Healing for Beginners'. Next we'll add a few more tools to your tool set in a chapter entitled 'Miscellaneous Reiki Exercises'.

10

REIKI - FULL 12 MERIDIAN HEALING

Here is a list of exercises that can help you help you in learning the Meridians. We've taken 12 exercises and turned them into one large exercise, so that you can learn and practice all 12 of the Meridians for Reiki healing. For best results, record yourself speaking so that you can play it back with music and give yourself a fully guided meditation, something that you can practice to ensure the memorization of the proper median points. Once you've learned these, combining them with the tradition based Reiki healing means that you can perform a healing that seems both simple and graceful, yet contains enough visualization and understanding of the human body in the background that it will prove effective. Don't expect to learn this overnight, it will take some time and patience, but we are certain that you'll be happy with the results. Let's now continue to the full Reiki healing so that you can learn your Meridians and go from there.

Reiki Yin and Yang Meridians - Full Healing

This is a full Reiki healing that you can perform as practice or as a form of 'preventative maintenance' to ensure that all of your Meridians are balanced. Record yourself reading it if you like and play a little music while your own voice walks you through the healing if you like. It's an excellent way to learn while encouraging good health in the body.

*Note: In this healing we are going to encompass all of your Meridians

1. Begin your breathing exercises. Focus on the counts of your breath until you become deeply and comfortably relaxed.

2. Place you hand, open palmed and fingers slightly spread, and place your hand just over your Heart so that you may access the Pericardium.

3. Draw Focus on your Chi. See it burning brightly around you, a white light that surrounds and fills you with joy and warmth. This same energy is in everyone and everything. It's you and it's the Universe. Take a moment to enjoy it's warmth and then we shall continue when you're ready.

4. Now that you're ready, draw excess Chi energy from your Pericardium. See it as a white light, almost to brilliant to look into, flowing into your hand, taking the form of a sphere. The first of the Yin and Yang pairings that we'll be healing are the Spleen and the Stomach. The Spleen is the Yin of this pairing, the Stomach is the Yang.

Yin and Yang 1 -The Spleen and the Stomach Meridians

5. Move your hand* down to your foot, placing it just over the outside edge of your big toe. This is the beginning of your Spleen Meridian. From here, move your palm from here up the inside of your legs, seeing the ball of light getting slowly smaller as the line of the Meridian illuminates and energizes. See the Meridian brightening as the Chi sphere passes through it. Move the light up your leg and to your thigh, passing further up to your abdomen. The ball of light should be dwindled to at least three-quarters, the Meridian glowing brightly where you've already touched it with the light. Take the light up further to the outside of the nipple and up to your second rib. The light orb is smaller now, most of the Meridian glowing brightly. Now, take the light to the terminus of the Meridian, the 6th space between your ribs. Take a moment to contemplate the entire illuminated Spleen Meridian and when you're ready we shall continue.

*Note: If you're already familiar with all of the Meridians, you don't need to trace your palm over the path that the lines take, but can instead keep your hand on the Pericardium to draw forth the excess Chi and visualize the ball of energy travelling over the Meridian lines.

6. Move your hand back to your Pericardium and draw more excess Chi into your hand. Don't worry about running out... Chi is around you, inside you, and pervades the Universe and every living thing. When you've gathered the energy into a glowing white ball, let's continue and heal the Stomach Meridian.

7. Move your hand and your healing light of Chi up to your face, moving it just under the center of your eye. This is where the Meridian of your Stomach begins. Move your hand down to the very edge of your jaw, seeing the Meridian line brighting as you pass the

light through it. Move your open palm slowly down your throat, almost touching but not quite, as the glowing orb feeds the Meridian and grows slowly smaller, continuing down to your abdomen and further down across the front of your leg.

Move the ball of light, now just a fraction of it's previous size, all the way down to your foot where the last of the light is absorbed at the terminus of the Meridian, the nail of your second toe. Take a moment to see the Meridian in its entirety, glowing brightly from the excess Chi that you've pushed there to imbalance and clear it of blockage. Once you've contemplated the Stomach Meridian then we can move on to the next pairing.

8. Move your hand, palm open and fingers lightly spread so that it's place over your Pericardium. Gather energy as before from your excess Chi, willing it into the shape of a ball of light hovering beneath your palm. We'll now 'trace' and heal the next two Meridians.

Yin and Yang 2 - The Lungs and The Large Intestine Meridians

9. Now we are going to heal the Yin of this pairing, the Lungs. Move your hand up close to your shoulder to the first space between your ribs. This is called the intercostal space and it's the starting point of the Lung Meridian. See the Meridian line flaring up as you pass the orb over it.

Move it up to the shoulder and down the front of your arm, the energy slowly transferring from the sphere of light in your palm as the Meridian is energized, dwindling to nothing as you take it down to the terminus of this Meridian, the fingernail of your thumb. Take a moment to admire the Lung Meridian, blazing brightly to your heightened senses. When you're ready, let's continue.

10. Move your hand back to your Pericardium and draw more excess Chi into your hand.

11. The Yang of the pairing is the Meridian of your Large Intestine. Move your open palm to your opposite hand to the beginning of this Meridian, the fingernail of your index finger. See the line shining as you direct the Chi energy in your hand to it and bring the light up your arm, tothe back of your shoulder, the ball of light becoming smaller as it's energy expends to balance and unblock this Meridian.

From the back of your shoulder, bring your hand up to your face to the terminus of this Meridian, your nostrils. Take a moment to observe the shining trail that the Large Intestine Meridian travels through your body and commit it to memory. When you're ready to continue we can go on to the next step.

12. Move your hand back to your Pericardium and draw more excess Chi into your hand.

Yin and Yang 3 - The Liver and the Gall Bladder Meridians

13. The Yin of our next pairing is the Liver. Move your open palm down to your foot and to our large toe. The Meridian begins just under the nail. See it lighten up with crackling, white Chi energy as you bring the orb to it's beginning. Move the orb in your hand slowly up your inner leg, moving next to your thigh.

See the energy dwindling, the orb shrinking slowly as you move along, the Meridian growing brighter as you pass. From the thigh, bring the light up the outside of your abdomen to it's terminus, your Sternum. Admire the newly illuminated path of the Liver Meridian for a moment to better commit it to memory and when you're ready, let's continue.

14. Move your hand back to your Pericardium and draw more excess Chi light into your hand.

15. The Yang of this pairing is the Gall Bladder. Let's heal this Meridian now. Move your hand up your face to the starting point of this Meridian, the outer corner of your eye. Visualize the start of the Meridian line flaring up as it greets the energy you're putting into it and will the Chi orb inside of your head and downward, where your hand will meet it at the front of your shoulder.

From here pass it down to your abdomen, noting how the orb is slowly dwindling as the Meridian grows brighter where it has been touched. Keep moving your hand down but release the orb to go inside of your abdomen, when it goes further down the Meridian at the bottom of your abdomen. Take the orb down the outer side of your leg to your foot and the Meridian's terminus, the nail or your fourth toe. Take a moment of contemplation to commit it to memory and then we shall move on. to the next pairing.

16. Move your hand once more to your Pericardium and collect more Chi energy.

Yin and Yang 4 - The Kidneys and the Bladder Meridians

17. The Yin of this pairing is the Kidneys Meridian. Move your hand down to the sole of your foot where this Meridian begins. See the Meridian flaring to life as you release some of the Chi energy into it. Move the Chi orb up the inside of your leg, noting as it slowly gets smaller and the Meridian brightens.

From the inside of your leg, move the light upwards to your abdomen and up further still to the terminus of this Meridian, the Clavicle. Take a moment to observe the brightened and empowered Meridian and commit it's path to memory and then we shall continue.

Collect more Chi energy from your Pericardium.

18. The Yang of this pairing is your Bladder. Move your Chi orb up to your face to the start of this Meridian, the inner-corner of your eye. Move the light over the top of your head and down your back (if not limber, you can visualize the orb moving by itself down your back). See it dwindling as it expends power slowly, causing the Meridian to crackle with energy as you move it further still, down your leg, li

Kidneys (Yin) and Bladder (Yang)

Bladder: This Meridian starts at the inner corner of your eye, where it then goes over the top of your head, moving down your back and leg until it terminates at the toenail of your pinky (smallest toe), absorbing the orb completely at last and leaving behind it a glowing trail that's your Bladder Meridian.

Take a moment to appreciate this line of power that the Ancients hold in such esteem. Commit to memory what you can and let's continue with the next pairing after charging up.

19. Gather a ball of healing energy from your Pericardium.

Yin and Yang 5 - The Heart and the Small Intestine

20. The Yin of this pairing is the Heart Meridian. It starts in your arm pit, so move your hand there and ignite the Meridian with the Chi energy that you've gathered in your hand. See it flaring up in response and bring the light further along the Meridian, down your inner arm and to your hand as the ball quickly dwindles and feeds energy into this shining line until finally expending itself at the terminus, your smallest finger. Take a moment to admire and memorize this simple, yet oh-so-important Meridian.

21. Move your hand over your Pericardium, palm-open and fingers outstretched slightly as you collect more excess Chi for the next step.

22. The Yang of this pairing is your Small Intestine Meridian. To begin, move your empowered hand to your opposite hand, placing it over the beginning of this Meridian, your smallest finger. See the Meridian brightening as you activate it like a circuit with your Chi energy.

Move your hand up the Meridian by taking it along the back of your arm, watching the energy dwindle slowly as you bring it up to your shoulder. Watch the orb, growing smaller as the Meridian grows brighter while you bring it down the shoulder, then up to your neck, finally moving it to its terminus, your ear, where it swallows the last of the energy. Take a moment to commit the path of this Meridian to memory and then we are ready to continue to the last pairing.

23. Move your hand to the Pericardium, with your palm open and held barely above the spot. Pull the excess Chi energy and shape it into a ball of healing white light.

Yin and Yang 6 - The Pericardium and the Triple Warmer

24. The Pericardium is the Yin of this pairing. Move your hand to the outside of the nipple in order to touch the Chi light to this location, as

it's the beginning of this Meridian. See the Meridian responding to the energy that the orb provides it.

From here, move the orb up your shoulder, seeing it becoming slightly smaller as the Meridian becomes brighter and you pass it down the front of your arm and to your hand. See the orb of light, tiny now. become absorbed as you reach the Meridian's terminus, your middle-finger. See the Meridian, bright and shining now and note the path for when you need it next time.

25. Gather up more excess Chi from your newly cleansed and empowered Pericardium, shaping the energy into a ball for the last portion of our healing.

26. The Triple Warmer is the Yang of this pairing and it's fitting that we do this last. As we've mentioned, this Meridian is important in that it governs your metabolism, body heat, and distribution of liquids throughout the entire body. After any healing is done this Meridian should be healed as well in case of imbalance or blockage from the Meridian that was blocked.

To heal this Meridian, move your open palm over the nail of your ring finger. See the Meridian respond, flaring to life as you bring the healing light up your forearm and continue up, the light sphere slowly growing smaller as the Meridian grows brighter as you move it to the back of your shoulder. From here, bring the light up to your ear and let its remaining energy all be absorbed at the terminus of this Meridian, your eyebrow.

27. Take a moment to contemplate the Triple Warmer Meridian, as well as all of the others which we've worked with in this healing.

Do you have all of the Meridians committed to memory yet? Keep practicing and soon you'll know them by heart. Good job, and consider this healing a success!

You've learned the Meridians. We can only give you the wisdom and knowledge. what you do with it's up to you. Take some time, let it soak in, learn every pathway, know your body, know your mind, know what the ancients wanted you to know. A system so old, you should take in the best of it and improve your understanding. Take the path of wisdom. You've come this far, why not go farther?

HEALING STONES TO INCORPORATE INTO REIKI AND CHAKRA HEALINGS

The following is a list of stones in the colors of your 7 Chakra points. These can be incorporated into healings by the placement of the appropriate color stones on its corresponding Chakra point before beginning the Reiki healing. Procure one or many of each color to add their natural influences while you're stimulating the Chakras and ensuring a more patient-specific healing session when you're performing Reiki. If needed, feel free to loan out stones with specific properties after a healing or acquire extra for distribution to patients. The results from adding these stones to your healings can be quite satisfying.

RED STONES: 1. RHODONITE

Healing Properties: Possessed of a lovely rose hue, this stone is famous for its properties in emotional healing. This is one that you'll definitely want to add to your collection. This silicate is good for calming anger and for the healing of traumas as well. Find it, add it to your healing toolbox.

2. Rose Quartz

Healing Properties: A powerful healer of the Heart both spiritually and physically, Rose Quartz can help you to open yourself emotionally when you've been wounded in the past. It also promotes a healthy circulatory system and strengthens your Heart. It's also very easy to obtain a nice piece for yourself, so be sure to add this to your collection soon.

3. Ruby

Healing Properties: Revered long by the ancients, legend has it that Kublai Khan once offered a city in exchange for a sizeable and apparently quite exquisite specimen. Thankfully in this day and age, you can obtain your own Ruby for quite a bit less (especially if purchased raw). Ruby inspires a vigor of the spirit and the body, driving one to live more fully. It can also assist with sexual dysfunction, fever, and constriction of the blood vessels. Star Ruby is said to have the same healing qualities, but magnified.

4. Bloodstone

Healing Properties: Bloodstone is good for detoxification and grounding negative energy. In matters of the heart it can help to ground negativity as well so this is a good stone to keep close.

5. Garnet

Healing Properties: Known as a simulator of creativity, Garnet is also a stone of sensuality, inciting passion into your love life and keepings things fresh.

6. Red Coral

Healing Properties: Strengthening circulation, as well as healing of the kidneys and the bladder, this stone pushes even further and assists in overall regeneration. The stone that grows like a plant can serve you well. Red Coral also acts as a natural antidepressant, so consider it for your healing toolbox.

ORANGE STONES: 1. SPESSARTINE GARNET

Healing Properties: Sometimes called 'the Garnet of the Sun', Spessartine Garnet can boost creativity as well as enhance cognitive function in matters of logic. This is a good stone to have when you're looking to make a life change as well, as the stone's energies are well aligned in that regard.

2. Orange Sunstone

Healing Properties: Nurturing feelings of generosity, the Orange Sunstone also empowers those who have lost a loved one with needed strength to weather the separation and move on. This stone also has a balancing and cleansing effect on all of the Chakras. This is also an excellent stone to have for empowering yourself against phobias through its joyful nature.

3. Carnelian

Healing Properties: Good for arthritis, lower back problems, and issues with the kidneys, Carnelian is also a good stone to have for stabilizing in the wake of an abusive relationship. It promotes accelerated healing and is also good for dealing with depression.

4. Orange Agate

Healing Properties: Orange Agate is an emotional stabilizer. Helping to keep you grounded, this is a good stone for anger management as well as for avoiding impulse decisions.

5. Orange Sapphire

Healing Properties: Orange Sapphire is a good stone for Artists and Writers, inspiring creativity. Use this to dispel writer's block or other issues of stifled creativity.

6. Orange Citrine

Healing Properties: Orange citrine is a promotes cognition. Physically, it helps to cleanse the kidneys, aids in digestion, detoxifies the blood and balances the thyroid. This is another good addition to your collection.

7. Amber

Healing Properties: Aiding in physical regeneration, Amber also acts as a natural purifier. Good for chronic pain, Amber also has a cleansing effect on all of the Chakra points. Amber is also reputed to draw sickness and disease from the body as well, due to its purification properties

8. Hessonite Garnet

Healing Properties: Hessonite Garnet is a powerful stone for treating ailments of the mind. Providing clarity of thought and confidence in the face of one's fears.

YELLOW STONES: 1. IRON PYRITE (ALSO CALLED FOOL'S GOLD)

Healing Properties: Acting as a powerful shield from negative energies, Iron Pyrite also enhances memory and is good for the healing of bones, reduction in swelling, and conditions of the lungs.

2. Yellow Citrine

Healing Properties: Good for anxiety, Yellow Citrine also acts as an amplifier for energies. This stone also aids in the treatment of eye issues as well, which empowering your lower 3 Chakras and your Third Eye Chakra as well.

3. Canary Yellow Tourmaline

Healing Properties: Canary Yellow Tourmaline works as a powerful mental stabilizer, as such it's good for anxiety, phobias, and can even help with Bipolar disorder. This stone can balance all of the Chakras as well so it's a good one to have around for your collection.

4. Gold

Healing Properties: Gold is good for a number of healing applications. For one, it acts as a natural amplifier to any minerals that it's paired with. Healing-wise, gold is said to help with issues such as the treatment of the nervous system, breathing issues, rejuvenation of the endocrine system and regeneration of tissue.

5. Lemon Quartz

Healing Properties: Lemon Quartz has a number of uses, including resistance to food and nicotine cravings, faster recovery following surgery, and promoting clarity of thought.

6. Yellow Sapphire

Healing Properties: Yellow Sapphires healing qualities tend more towards the spiritual, as it encourages one to turn creativity into action. As such it can be used to inspire and break through creative blocks or other hindrances in life.

7. Crysoberyl

Healing Properties: Crysoberyl is good for healing of chest and liver issues. It's also good for skin problems, digestion issues, balancing the adrenal glands, and has a positive effect regarding the balance of cholesterol in your body.

8. Golden Beryl

Healing Properties: Opening the Purple and Yellow Chakras, Golden Beryl is good for achieving a calm and peaceful state of emotions. This is a good stone to have when recovering from mental trauma as it can help to soothe the weary spirit.

GREEN STONES: 1. GREEN AVENTURINE

Healing Properties: Good for the lungs, heart, the sinuses, and the liver, this is an excellent stone to include in an intensive healing session. This stone is also said to enhance creativity.

2. Chrysoprase

Healing Properties: Stimulating your Orange and Green Chakras, Chrysoprase healing your inner child or a broken heart. Phsycially, it acts as a strong detoxifier for the liver and combats insomnia for a restful and good nights sleep.

3. Serpentine

Healing Properties: An excellent stone to include in Reiki healings, Serpentine assists in the directing of healing energies. Another detoxifier, Serpentine can help in cleansing toxins from your body and also helps in treating hypoglycemia.

4. Hiddenite

Healing Properties: This stone is good for deep emotional healing, such as for victims of abuse, addition, or those in the severe throes of grief for a lost loved one.

5. Jade

Healing Properties: Jade is good for conditions of the Spleen, the Kidneys, and the Bladder. It also boosts mental access to the spiritual world and inspires creativity.

6. Peridot

Healing Properties: Revered by Egyptian kings to the extent that touching one without permission was grounds for death, the Peridot is good for treating tobacco and other addictions. Especially prized for Reiki healing, the Peridot can help in guiding your hands as well as for recovery of energies after healings.

7. Chalcedony

Healing Properties: Good for the healing of bones, your circulatory system, eyes, and your spleen, Chalcedony is a good multifunction healer to add to your collection of healing stones.

8. Green Agate

Healing Properties: Green agate is primarily used for bringing the body and mind back into harmony. Emotionally it's good for dealing with repressed anger and fears, due to the calming influence exerted by the stone.

9. Green Garnet

Healing Properties: Encouraging regeneration and growth, this stone also increases vitality and promotes an air of compassion when dealing with others.

10. Amazonite

Healing Properties: Amazonite enhances communication, imparting the ability to see things from the point of view of others. This stone is good for healing creative blocks and for opening the closed mind.

11. Green Apatite

Healing Properties: Enhancing hand and eye coordination, Green Apatite is useful for healing in that it helps to maintain a good and stable energy flow at the same time that it's stimulating your Green Chakra.

12. Emerald

Healing Properties: Emerald is good for invigorating thought and useful in the treatment of a damaged memory. It's also good for reviving passions in one who has suffered from abuse or addiction and is seeking to enjoy life anew.

BLUE STONES: 1. AQUAMARINE

Healing Properties: Good for hormonal issues, throat problems, Thyroid issues, and swollen glands, Aquamarine is a good stone to have in your healing collection.

2. Labradorite

Healing Properties: Good for detoxification from alcohol or tobacco, this stone also helps to stabilize more negative aspects of our personalities, such as anger, envy, jealousy, and such.

3. Blue Lace Agate

Healing Properties: This stone opens and clears the Throat Chakra, as well as promoting energies that help you to destroy old patterns and modes of thinking that have proven destructive in your current life.

4. Aragonite

Healing Properties: Stimulating the Green, Blue, and Indigo Chakras, this stone promotes communication and healing from past traumas. It also amplifies empathy, which can prove quite useful for healers.

5. Blue Apatite

Healing Properties: A creativity enhancer, this stone also promotes hunger suppression so it can be useful for those trying to lose weight.

6. Celestine

Healing Properties: Another creativity stimulator, this stone is also good for dispelling anxiety. It's also attuned to the celestial and can increase the strength of guidance for the hand positions employed in Reiki healings.

7. Benetoite

Healing Properties: A stimulator of the Indigo Chakra, this stone is good for lethargy, imparting energy to get through the day for those who find themselves always tired.

8. Azurite

Healing Properties: Azurite is a stone that stimulates all of the mind, making it a good healer for those who are feeling burnt-out or who find themselves stuck in a cycle of despair.

9. Blue Topaz

Healing Properties: Stimulating the Indigo Chakra as well as the Blue Chakra, this stone can help to heal phobias associated with public speaking, boosting confidence and communication abilities.

10. Blue Aventurine

Healing Properties: This is a stone that asserts willpower for overcoming negative habits. Use it for assistance in quitting smoking, overcoming anger, substance abuse, and more. This stone can impart that additional 'oomph.' that you need to get the job done.

11. Turquoise

Healing Properties: Considered sacred by the Native Americans and other cultures, such as the Tibetans and early Egyptians, this stone has a number of properties. Good for the immune system, your bones, and for detoxifying the body, this stone also assists in effective communication with others.

12. Blue Sapphire

Healing Properties: Another stone that grants guidance of the hands, this stone is popular with Reiki healers. A stone of love, Sapphire can impart understanding of higher ideals and help to suppress feelings of powerlessness and break blocks from a focus that has been reduced to the micro level from extreme traumas in life.

INDIGO STONES

1. Indigo Crystal

Healing Properties: Indigo crystals are the perfect stone for focusing self examination, a detachment of thought that explores the possibilities as envisioned from the minds of others. Use these in healing someone who clings too hard to ego. If they're sensitive, then advise that it's a stone for empathy, not all are ready to divorce their ego for truth.

2. Indigo Labradorite

Healing Properties: This stone assists with disorders of the mind and of the eyes. This stone works with the Triple Warmer, regulating metabolism and hormones. Keep this stone handy for imparting power in the closing healings of your Reiki sessions.

3. Iolite

Healing Properties: A motivator, Iolite restores perspective. This is a strong stone to incorporate into healings where there are issues with one's family.

4. Tanzanite

Healing Properties: Strengthening te Indigo Chakra, this stone can assist in empowering intuition. This stone is best used when fueling a burnt-out sense of spirituality.

5. Crystal Sodalite

Healing Properties: Assisting with calcium deficiencies, this stone can also quicken the immune system, as well as functioning as a metabolism booster. A good stone to have handy.

VIOLET STONES: 1. VIOLET SODALITE

Healing Properties: Encouraging rational though, Violet sodalite also helps in preventing panic attacks.

2. Amethyst

Healing Properties :Inducing calm, this stone is paramount in matters of the nervous system. This stone is also strong in strengthening relationships.

3. Violet Topaz

Healing Properties: Recharges all of the Meridians and aids in spiritual insight.

4. Violet Beryl

Healing Properties: Provides a magnification effect to healings, this is a must-have for the more serious practitioners.

5. Violet Tourmaline

Healing Properties: Reducing fear, this stone breaks creativity blocks and pushes overall happiness.

6. Jadeite

Healing Properties: Protecting against fatigue, enhancing the circulatory system, and empowering longevity, think of this as the 'long life' stone.

7. Spinel

Healing Properties: Revitalization in the face of challenges, this stone helps the recipient to deal with problems as they would in youth and power. Providing a fount of seemingly endless energy, this is the stone for the conquering of will over want.

8. *Violet apatite*

Healing Properties: Enhancing the Blue Chakra, this stone sharpens communication to a level tat is almost the poet. Use sparingly, sometimes people react poorly to the world described with accuracy, especially the personal world.

9. *Barite*

Healing Properties: Energy alignment and spiritual focus, this is for those who are ready to progress.

AFTERWORD

You've learned about Meridians, standard Reiki, and gone well on your path for healing others and self-healing. We've gone into Mantras and Chakra points, in order to ensure that you not only have the basics, but that you're educated in what you need to know to get started effectively.

Be sure to practice the Meridians, learn the Traditional hand placements, and then take that knowledge and build from there. Once you've done the healing exercises a number of times and once you've seen the results then we are certain that you'll be happy with the fruits of your labor.

Now you've started you Reiki journey, you'll find it will lead you to new insights, discoveries, body-mind healing techniques, and even new people and places. Reiki is spreading rapidly around the world and we are constantly learning more about its profound healing capabilities, so make sure you continue to practice and deepen your knowledge in this wonderful ancient art of healing.

Peace and blessings to you all,

Siya Ishani

www.ingramcontent.com/pod-product-compliance
Lightning Source LLC
Chambersburg PA
CBHW071858070526
44583CB00016B/1753